Developmental
Disorders of Language

Second Edition

Catherine Adams, Betty Byers Brown
and Margaret Edwards

W
Whurr Publishers Ltd
London

© 1997 Whurr Publishers Ltd
First published 1997 by
Whurr Publishers Ltd
19b Compton Terrace, London N1 2UN, England

Reprinted 1999 and 2001

British Library Cataloguing in Publication Data
A catalogue record for this book is available from the
British Library.

ISBN: 1 86156 020 6

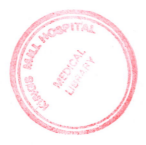

Printed and bound in the UK by Athenaeum Press Ltd,
Gateshead, Tyne & Wear

Contents

Contents

Preface to the Second Edition

Since the publication of the first edition of this book we have suffered the very sad loss of one of the authors, Betty Byers Brown. Every effort has been made to preserve the intent and spirit of her contribution and the original format is unchanged. The necessary updating has resulted in some deletions to take account of changes which have taken place over the last seven years. In particular chapter eight has been extended and rewritten so that it addresses more comprehensively the problems now confronting those concerned with children's language disorders. The complexities of identification, diagnosis and terminology have also been discussed at greater length so as to reflect current views.

We are indebted to Dr Hilary Gardner who is responsible for the updating of chapters four and six. Jennifer Warner's and Anne Hesketh's help and advice are very much appreciated. Jennifer and Anne are colleagues of Catherine Adams, who has succeeded Betty Byers Brown as my co-author.

Margaret Edwards
London 1997

Note
To avoid the use of he/she and mother/father, the child has been referred to as he and the parent as mother throughout the book.

Chapter 1
Characterisation

Summary

This chapter describes those children who have developmental disorders of language and indicates how they may present to the lay public and to the professional. It discusses how the term 'developmental language disorder' has come to supersede earlier terminologies. Estimates of prevalence, drawn from the literature of both speech impairment and language disability, are given. A theoretical network is introduced within which language disorders in developing children may be considered. The pervasive nature of language disorder is emphasised together with its relationship to later learning disabilities. This introduction paves the way for the specific processes of identification and management that are discussed in subsequent chapters.

Who are these children?

Children with developmental language disorders are those who are unable to communicate effectively through language or to use language as a basis for learning. They are handicapped socially, educationally and, as a natural consequence, emotionally. Their handicap has been described as an invisible one because it is not obvious to the casual observer. There are no cosmetic or prosthetic signs to suggest that something is amiss. In the park, the playground or the shopping mall a language-disordered child may be indistinguishable from his normal peers. It is only the discerning observer or the professional who may see indications that the child is not fully equipped to take his place among his peers or that he is abnormally ill at ease in a social situation. Such indications include distress in a noisy or swiftly speaking environment; excessive restlessness or impulsivity; immature and dependent behaviour; poor motor coordination; inappropriate speech or reluctance to make communicative contact, particularly with strangers. These signs may alert the informed but will not carry the message to the casual passer-by.

1

The 'lay person' may first suspect that something is wrong when he or she tries to engage the child in conversation or makes some overture to which speech would be a natural response. The actual response may be withdrawal or refusal, inappropriate clinging to the parent who may appear over-protective or else a reply in speech that the person making the overture may fail to understand. This person may react with affront or embarrassment and yet another situation has been created in which the child feels inadequate and the parent ashamed or annoyed. The accumulation of inadequacies as the result of these encounters may have a profound effect upon the child's emotional well-being. If he is also being exposed to continuous failure at school, the effect will be compounded. School failure is difficult to avoid where there is language disorder because the child is unable to master the structure of his native language or to use that language creatively and flexibly. He may have reading and writing difficulties in addition to his impaired oral communication. In view of the heavy emphasis placed upon language in so many aspects of the school curriculum and the fact that ability to comprehend language underpins so many learning tasks, it will be difficult for a teacher to find a subject in which the language-disordered child can excel.

The 'speech and language therapist in practice' will encounter developmental language disorder in all its manifestations at every stage of the child's development. A very familiar introduction is through the child who presents with delayed speech. A typical referral is that of a child, usually male, of between 2;6 and 3 years of age who uses a few words and no connected utterances. Hearing tests reveal no impairment of acuity; psychological assessment suggests that cognitive functioning is within normal limits. It will then fall upon the speech and language therapist to establish whether or not the delay in speech reflects a more serious disorder in the ability to acquire language. If so, some indication must be given as to future educational needs in addition to those of language therapy. The immediate course of action may involve therapy for the child and guidance for the parents.

Alternatively, the young child may appear in the clinic with equivocal responses to sound and speech and failure to comprehend spoken language. Again, the course will be one of investigation and prediction combined with immediate guidance and support. Other referrals may include school-aged children who appear to be unable to organise their spoken language in a coherent and fluent manner; those who are experiencing reading difficulties which appear to be related to their understanding and use of language; and children who have not eradicated early speech problems that now appear to have another basis than simple immaturity. These children will require full diagnostic, linguistic assessment and a programme of remediation by therapist and teacher.

The 'speech and language therapist in training' may encounter any of the cases mentioned above while carrying out practical work in a community clinic. Or, the first experience with developmental language disorders may be through visiting a language unit. In this case the student will look for some common denominator among the children. In a pre-school unit this is likely to be delayed speech. It may be manifest in immature syntax, poor vocabulary or a restricted or unstable phonological system. The student may also be impressed by the children's poor level of attention, particularly with regard to listening. Further observation may reveal a relative poverty of symbolic play and deficiencies in behaviours such as turn-taking, which normally precede communication through language.

If the first encounter with developmental language disorder comes about through visits to a regular primary or junior school for purposes of classroom observation, the child with a language disorder may appear to constitute a class of one. Beveridge and Conti-Ramsden (1987), give some indication of the range of behaviours that may be encountered: unintelligible speech; simple or limited expressive language; withdrawal and non-participation; inability to see a joke; literal mindedness; attention problems. It is only after considerable acquaintance with the process of language development that it is possible to begin to see how these behaviours may be united. The failure to master the basic underpinnings of language at an early age means that the skill may never be used with assurance and exactitude even though many of its components may eventually be mastered.

Byers Brown (1971) pointed out the one characteristic that such children might have in common. Describing a group of language-disordered pupils gathered together for a summer-school programme she observed 'They showed all kinds of learning and behaviour problems which seemed to stem from their disordered and confused speech' (p. 85). With these problems were associated inattention, idiosyncratic spelling and poor physical coordination. *'The one thing that they had in common was an obvious and pervasive sense of failure.'*

The sense of failure may be much less apparent once such children are placed in an educational environment where their needs are understood and the curriculum adapted to allow for full participation by all members of the class. Within a special school of this kind, the atmosphere should be buoyant and hopeful and the children lively and communicative. There are very few schools in the UK that cater specifically for the language-disordered and these schools are highly selective as to which children they admit. They tend to receive those children with very severe disorders who cannot be managed within a local education system. Such children may have to be taught an alternative language system because spoken language may prove impracticable as a means of communication and systematic instruction. A person visiting such a school would receive a very different impression of 'language disorder' from that gained in any of the other situations described.

There are several professions that share responsibility for the care and management of language-disordered children but that of speech and language therapy demands the most continuous involvement. This is because so many disorders of language manifest themselves through delayed and disordered speech. It is also because the title 'speech and language therapist' carries the connotation of involvement in all areas of language failure or breakdown. This responsibility means that language - disordered children place severe demands upon a speech and language therapy service. This is not due to sheer weight of numbers for, indeed, these have yet to be properly estimated. Rather it is due to the nature and course of language disorders that manifest themselves in many different ways and at different times. As a consequence, there is need for both flexibility and continuity in service provision and, where services are scantily funded and staffed, these requirements are difficult to meet and to maintain.

Children with developmental disorders of language do not constitute the only group with difficulty in acquiring language. Among the others are those who suffer from hearing impairment, intellectual handicap or autism. Children who are socially disadvantaged may lack the opportunity to experience language in all its richness and so they may be slow to master it and use it with ease. Children with cerebral palsy, who are severely restricted in movement, may be unable to experience the full range of language. They will be limited in their use of it as a tool even though they may be capable of mastering its basic structure. When there is more than one handicap, as in the case of a hearing-impaired child in an emotionally and socially impoverished home, the difficulties are, of course, compounded. In all these cases, the language handicap is secondary to another condition and would not have arisen in its absence.

Table 1.1 shows in summary form some characteristic cases of language-disordered children as they present to the speech and language therapist.

What is a developmental language disorder?

The broad term 'developmental language disorder' simply denotes that something has gone wrong with the language behaviour of the developing child. It is a descriptive term that covers a range of conditions and impairments from word-finding difficulty to the inability to generate and maintain personal and social relationships through language. Bloom and Lahey (1978) used the term as a descriptive label. They believed it to be necessary to use the term descriptively rather than diagnostically in order to refer to a range of behaviours without making a specific diagnosis on aetiological grounds or one that could imply permanent incapacity. As used currently, it covers all manner of deficits in oral comprehension and expression together with impairments of the written word.

Table 1.1 Characteristic cases of developmental language disorder

Age at referral (years)	Sex	Presenting symptom	History	Findings	Recommendations	Progress
2;6	M	Failure to produce words	Normal development apart from late sitting	Hearing and non-verbal intelligence normal; play limited and stereotyped	Language therapy and parent guidance	Very slow acquisition of all expressive language; problems persisting in articulatory precision
2;11	F	Failure to combine words	History unremarkable apart from head circumference in 90th percentile to height and weight in 50th percentile No neurological disorder	Hearing and cognitive development normal emotional maturity	Language monitoring and parent guidance	Steady growth in syntax and language use Phonology slow to develop but normal by 7 years
3;2	M	No sentences	Threatened abortion at 3 months but carried to term Born with cord around neck Late walking and clumsy; daytime enuresis, nail biting and hair pulling	Hearing within normal limits; wide scatter of ability shown on non-verbal intelligence; perceptuomotor problems	Language therapy	Language and learning difficulties persisting into junior school
2;6	M	No speech	Delivered by caesarean section because of placenta praevia Birthweight 9 lb 7 oz Milestones slightly delayed: sitting 10/12; walking 19/12	Responded to distraction testing at 40–60 dB	Further investigation and parent guidance Subsequent findings suggested auditory processing difficulty and conductive loss Medical treatment improved hearing but poor auditory skills persisted	Persisting difficulty with comprehension and expression of language; word-finding difficulty

As a generic class, developmental language disorder includes those few conditions that present as clearly definable and identifiable syndromes such as 'verbal auditory agnosia' (Rapin and Allen, 1983, 1987) and a much larger group of loosely classified behaviours such as 'language delay'. The term has emerged and established itself because of its clinical utility and its popularity is enhanced by its avoidance of controversial terminology. However, its use has done nothing to clarify the field that it represents. Schery (1985) reporting upon a major investigation of language-disordered children found it necessary to qualify the label by adding 'labelled variously developmentally aphasic, dysphasic, language impaired, specific language disabled and language delayed'.

Developmental language disorder has no single aetiology. It co-exists with and without demonstrable neurological impairment. Whilst closely associated with hearing loss, intellectual handicap, emotional disturbance and environmental deprivation, it cannot be wholly explained by them because it is found in children who are 'normal' in every other way. It may be better to consider the capacity of the child to develop language as being affected by a variety of deleterious factors, that might include any or all of the above, and a more circumscribed condition where, despite an adequate environment and intact modalities, the child inherits a predisposition to abnormal development of the neurological mechanisms underlying language (Bishop, 1992a).

In view of the complexity and diversity of the conditions grouped together under the broad heading of 'language disorder', it is not surprising to find that there were some reservations to the use of the term when first propounded on the grounds that it suggested a homogeneity that was not there to be found. Not only do the children in the group show different symptoms from each other but they have entered the group by different routes. Some are positively diagnosed as having a language disorder on the basis of tests constructed for the purpose. Others have been identified by exclusion: the child is not deaf; not intellectually retarded in the general sense; not autistic; not dysarthric and so must be language-disordered. Paul (1992) points out that the definition of developmental language disorders by exclusion arose from the writings of Benton (1964), but that the concept of an exclusive condition of language deficit has been understood for a century or more. Had we arrived at more positive forms of identification at a point coincident with our developing interest (i.e. in the 1960s and 1970s), the subsequent paths of both children and professionals would have been a great deal easier.

Is Specific Language Disorder different from developmental language disorder?

The need to disassociate language disorders from other handicapping conditions and affirm them as handicapping in their own right has led to the use of 'specific' as a qualifier (Stark and Tallal, 1981; Gordon, 1987; Ripley, 1987). Whilst this places the emphasis firmly upon language as the source of the handicap, it tends to make for clumsiness without improving clarity. It is used by some for conditions where there is a proven neurological basis for the condition and by others for conditions defined by the exclusion of all other pathologies. Robinson (1987) uses the term with reference to a special school population with widely varying prenatal, postnatal and perinatal aetiologies. To further complicate matters some authors provide definitions of 'developmental language disorders' that clearly might be another writer's definition of specific language impairment (SLI). For instance Cantwell and Baker (1987) define developmental language disorder as 'a disturbance or delay in language acquisition that is unexplained by general mental retardation, hearing impairment, neurological impairments or physical abnormalities'. Used with 'impairment' instead of 'disorder', the word 'specific' appears to have more exactitude, but we cannot assume that there is general agreement as to what constitutes this specific impairment. In a sense there is an interesting relationship between the difficulties of definition and the profile of impairment. For instance (with reference to Bloom and Lahey's model of language development, (Bloom and Lahey, 1978)), we might advocate that the term specific language impairment might be applied only to those children with deficits of language 'form', the so-called phonologic – syntactic disorder (see Chapter 5), and this seems to be the focus of much SLI research in the US. If impairments in content and use occur, then frequently they are associated with manifestations of social or intellectual impairments. But nothing is so precise in language disorders that such clear distinctions may be made, and content/use impairments *may* arise where there is no such explanatory aetiology, either as a conjunct or a result of the central language deficit.

To speak of language being disordered is to say nothing of the process that has brought it about. It is merely to give a name to a broad group of conditions that are related in so much as they affect language. It is useful to particularise the group even in such a broad way because it encourages us to examine the ways in which language that is disordered differs from language that is acquired in the normal manner and at a normal rate. It also prompts us to examine the ways in which language-disordered children differ from their normally developing peers without making aetiological assumptions. Nevertheless, it remains a broadly descriptive term to which the addition of the word 'specific' can only lend a spurious exactitude. Leonard (1987) concludes that the term 'specific language impairment' is of 'questionable value' with regard to empirical research, and may be irrelevant to service provision issues. It is quite possible that it is a term appropriate to this phase of our evolution of the subject, which will be discarded when the conditions that it covers have been more clearly identified. We may see a return to a more specific terminology but one that is supported by the clear delineation of clinical subtypes.

How prevalent is developmental language disorder?

Present estimates of the prevalence of developmental language disorder are likely to be less than accurate for the following reasons:

- The use of such terms as 'speech defect' and 'speech disorder' among early studies. These criteria have led to the acquisition of articulate speech being used as an outcome measure. As a consequence, the persistence of language difficulties has not been measured or represented accurately.
- The inclusion of a number of known pathologies such as cerebral palsy, cleft palate and autism. These conditions are associated with difficulties and delays in acquiring speech and/or language but their inclusion prevents proper estimate as to the number of children whose handicap is *restricted* to the area of language.
- The lack of appropriate measures by which to assess both normal and deviant language development at the time when early surveys were undertaken.
- The differences in expertise and professional viewpoints of those taking part in the surveys.
- The lack of distinction between children with true language deficit and those with delays attendant upon socio-economic status or cultural difference.

Unfortunately we cannot expect to gain a much clearer idea as to the numbers of children whose language abilities are impaired in relation to their other abilities until the field of language disorder is considerably clarified. The lack of conceptual clarity affects not only the way in which we treat these children but the way in which we identify and describe them. Berger (1987) points out that: 'epidemiological studies of partic-ular forms of disorder cannot proceed until the phenomena of interest have been defined in ways that enable them to be discriminated and measured. These definitions then give rise to particular estimates of prevalence and incidence and can influence service provision and plan-ning. Defined in other ways, different estimates may ensue'.

Nevertheless, in order to provide for language-disordered children in the immediate future, we have to make use of such figures as we have. Those surveys that are most frequently quoted will be presented and should be read with the above provisos in mind.

Surveys

A widely quoted survey is that undertaken by Morley and colleagues as part of a major study of 1000 families in Newcastle-upon-Tyne. The procedures and results as they pertain to speech development and disturbances and to early language development, are fully discussed by Morley in the original and revised texts of her classic work *The Development and Disorders of Speech in Childhood* (Morley, 1972). Morley reports a figure of 10% of children delayed in speech at 2 years of age, 6% at 3;9 and 3–5% at the time of school entry (4;9). She also records a figure of 3% with defects of speech and language at 6;6 years. Morley and her colleagues did not carry out detailed investigations into subsequent educational attainments so it is possible that some of her early speech delays did have persisting problems in associated areas of language. The fact that none of them was referred for special education is not necessarily significant.

Mac Keith and Rutter (1972) in their note on the prevalence of speech and language disorders state that 1% of children come to school with a marked language handicap and that a further 4–5% may show sequelae of early language difficulties. However, guidelines from the Association For All Speech Impaired Children (AFASIC, 1988) state that the 1972 estimate is considered to be 'a gross underestimate and should be used as an indicator only'.

Marge, also reporting in 1972, indicated a 6.2% prevalence of language disability in pupils between the ages of 4 and 17 years in the US population. Tuomi and Ivanoff (1977) give an estimate of 6–7% for language disabilities among a kindergarten population and first grade population of 900 in Canada. This figure receives some support from a later Canadian study that finds 8.04% of 5-year-old kindergarten children showing language problems (Beitcham et al., 1986).

Silva (1980) reviews a number of epidemiological studies and points out that the more recent ones have tended to focus on the pre-school child and particularly the 3-year-old. He considers this to be because language develops dramatically in the pre-school period. It could also be because investigators have more confidence in the measures that can be used at an early age because of our increased knowledge of early language development. If so, that confidence may be misplaced, certainly with regard to the stability of the findings. Many authors feel that it is not appropriate to use such terms as 'disability' or 'disorder' about the language of very young children because delay in acquisition may prove to be transient. Estimates of language delay in pre-school children do not necessarily distinguish between levels of delay. The following studies are those in which some distinctions are made.

Stevenson and Richman (1976) identified 3–4% of 705 3-year-old children as language delayed by at least 6 months. Fifty per cent of the children so delayed were generally retarded. Only four children had roughly normal cognitive ability in conjunction with significant language delay. Randall, Reynell and Curwen (1974) in a study of 300 3-year-olds found only one case of a specific, significant language delay that was still present at 4 years. The authors discuss this finding in relation to the prevalence figure of 1% yielded by other studies (Mac Keith and Rutter, 1972) and to the estimate range of 1–0.7% per 1000. They conclude that 'if, as seems likely, a true developmental language disorder occurs to approximately the same extent as other developmental disorders (i.e. not more than 1 to 2 per 1000)' (p. 15) then their sample, which was reduced by attrition to 160, 'was much too small'.

Fundudis, Kolvin and Garside (1979) found that, of 3300 Newcastle children, 4% were speech retarded in that they were not using words strung together to make sentences. This 4% was considered to be a conservative estimate. Their follow-up procedures revealed that 18 of the children could be classified under 'pathologically deviant'. One of these was classified as 'severe dysphasia' but the others were in non-linguistic pathological categories. The remaining 84 children were classified as having a 'residual speech handicap' and their prevalence estimate was about 2–3% of children of school age.

Silva (1980), reporting on his sample of 937 3-year-old children in New Zealand, gave a figure of 8% as being significantly delayed in either language expression (2%), language comprehension (3%) or both (3%). The most stable figure was that given for both comprehension and expression and this included a high percentage of children who were intellectually retarded or borderline.

In one of the few studies of 2-year-olds, Rescorla (1984) gives an estimate of 10% language delay. She explains the discrepancy between this figure and the percentage generally estimated for 3-year-olds (3–5%) by suggesting that some percentage of 2-year-olds will surely have developed normal speech by the age of 3. Rescorla's figure is based upon a sample of 351 children between the ages of 22 and 26 months. There is good agreement between her figures and Morley's early findings on delayed speech development, with the same argument of delayed maturation advanced by both. In a later paper Rescorla confirmed the findings of 10% prevalence in a 'middle-class' sample, but feels that the prevalence may well be higher in disadvantaged populations (Rescorla, 1989).

The report of Invalid Children's Aid Nationwide (ICAN, 1988) accepts a figure of 0.08 as the prevalence for 'specific language disorders' and points out that the prevalence of language disorders among the pre-school population is greater than for the school-aged population. This report makes clear distinction between language delay and language disorder. The bulk of the report is devoted to provision for school-aged children. Extrapolating from the findings of the 1972 paper (Mac Keith and Rutter, 1972) the authors estimate that the current UK population of school-aged children will contain approximately 5600 who are language-disordered. They estimate that 'it is generally accepted that the prevalence of language handicap decreases with age' (p. 4) more than half of the children will be between the ages of 5 and 11.

Enderby and Davies (1989) attempted to estimate from sample statistics the need for speech and language therapy for children with speech and language disorders. They estimated the rate of occurrence for the condition to be 968 per 100 000 children, between the ages of 3 and 9 years only.

We have no clear estimates of numbers of children who show reading or writing disorders later in school life as a symptom of continuing language disorder. However, the association between early language delay and disorder and subsequent learning disability is very strong (Strominger and Bashir, 1977; Aram and Nation, 1980; Silva, McGee and Williams, 1983; Snowling, 1987; Tallal, 1987). Longitudinal studies (e.g. Bishop and Adams, 1990) have shown convincing evidence for the consequences of early language impairment on reading comprehension skills and other studies, (Paul and Cohen, 1984; Stone, 1992), have demonstrated that the consequences of early deficits reach far into the social and emotional domains, which in turn have a negative impact on educational progress.

It is therefore possible that the 1% estimate will be revised. Even if it is not, this cold little statistic still represents a great deal in terms of human misery and wasted potential. Those in the remedial professions will find in it evidence enough to continue to revise and extend their skills on behalf of the language-disordered.

Speech and language therapists may deduce from such figures as we have, that they will have a responsibility towards all school-aged children with disordered language, which will occupy a considerable amount of corporate clinical time. It will almost certainly be exceeded by their involvement with pre-school children. They will be required to participate in investigations aimed at clarifying which delays are transient and which are associated with continuing disorders. They will be involved in programmes of guidance and prophylaxis and in individual therapy. Whatever the exact figures on language delay, it is continuously cited as the most common developmental problem found in pre-school children (Bax, Hart and Jenkins, 1980; Snyder-McClean and McClean, 1987).

The evolution of a terminology

One predictable consequence of a changing terminology is that it tends to suggest that a new group of children has been discovered. In some instances this is justified but the case of 'developmental language disorders' is not one of them. These children have been discussed and described for many years but under a number of different labels. A new label indicates either an increase in knowledge or a change in thinking or both. It should not prevent students and clinicians from studying cases labelled by other names or texts using different terminology. To do this would be to negate a great deal of professional knowledge. The following historical review will draw attention to the change in terminology and indicate how it reflects changes in thinking. To ponder on historical roots is not merely an academic exercise, but may assist in the clarification of current perspectives.

Developmental aphasia

The term 'developmental aphasia' may be found in the literature of language pathology from its inception and is well represented in the period from 1950 to 1970, and was then broadly used to describe children of normal intelligence who were failing to develop spoken language. The last text published in the UK under the name developmental dysphasia was that edited by Wyke in 1978. This text contains valuable and pertinent information for all those concerned with developmental language disorders. Chiat and Hirson (1987), select the term 'dysphasia' as being the most appropriate for the case under discussion in their paper. Stark and Tallal use the term frequently to describe their research subjects' condition (McCauley, 1988). The move away from general use of the term was part of the reconsideration of the receptive–expressive dichotomy that dominated the clinical language field and that owed its origins to the study of acquired aphasia in adults. Terminology based upon the receptive–expressive language model was current at the time when British speech and language therapists were starting to publish their findings. These added considerably to the sparse publications of the few neurologists and paediatricians who were interested in speech and language disorders. Conspicuous among speech and language therapists was the work of Morley (1960, 1973). Morley contributed a number of case studies on developmental aphasia and discussed how the condition might be differentiated from delayed speech. Cases of both receptive aphasia (with and without hearing loss) and expressive aphasia were cited. Expressive aphasia is illustrated in cases with and without cerebral palsy. Developmental aphasia is associated in all cases with neurological dysfunction but described in terms of delayed neurological maturation of the central processes involved.

Griffiths (1964, 1972) describes and discusses cases of both receptive and expressive developmental aphasia drawn from the records of the John Horniman School. This establishment, like its sister school, Moor House, was strongly influenced in its diagnostic determinations by the work of the medical director Worster-Drought. Worster-Drought's name is strongly associated with the condition of 'congenital auditory imperception' that he first identified (Worster-Drought and Allen, 1930). This condition is closely allied to Rapin's more recent 'verbal auditory agnosia' (a severe receptive language deficit). The inability of some children to recognise the meaning of speech sounds that both these terms represent, is continuously documented in the literature of both hearing and language disorders (Ingram, 1959; McGinnis, 1963; Morley, 1973; Ward and McCartney, 1978). The influence of Worster-Drought was recognised by a number of authors in the 1960s (Lea, 1965; Gordon, 1966; Thomas, 1969) including teachers, therapists and neurologists. Lea was one of the many workers at that time who also emphasised the symbolic nature of the aphasic disturbance in receptive aphasia.

Greene (1964) points out some of the ambiguities inherent in the term 'aphasia' as applied to developmental states. Many speech and language therapists then considered that there was sufficient similarity between the developmental and acquired adult condition for the same term to be used. This view was opposed by the neurologists. Some investigators therefore restricted their use of aphasia in childhood to the acquired state. Greene states that the term should never be used for delays in speech and language that are transcended by 5 or 6 years of age. However, she later indicated that there was no way of knowing which delays would recover by that time and which would not. One must deduce that the term 'aphasia' was not to be used until around 6 years of age when the delays were characterised as gross and persisting and carried a poor prognosis.

In the same paper Greene (1964) refers to the incomplete nature of investigations carried out into developmental aphasia, much of which she attributes to specialist bias. Representatives of different professions would look only for those signs that they perceived as significant. A notable example was that of the neurologists who would not take language delays seriously in the absence of clear or 'hard' neurological signs. Because the medical profession carried major responsibility for referring children for therapy and special education, this attitude was a source of considerable frustration to therapists and teachers as well as to parents. Although medical literature distinguished between 'developmental aphasia' and transient speech delays, there was no correspondence between the developmental aphasia group and those few children who showed sufficiently clear signs of neuropathology to satisfy the neurologists. *The term 'developmental aphasia' seemed thus to invite controversy while not assisting remediation.* It is not surprising that workers in the field became dissatisfied with it. Greene points out that many authorities preferred to use a term that could cover the range of speech delays and yet could also be used to refer to the severe and prolonged state of developmental aphasia. 'Developmental language disorder' accordingly started to replace 'developmental aphasia'.

The term 'language disorders' gained rapid popularity in the USA under such notable championship as that of Berry (1969). Berry propounds a concept of language behaviour that involves psychoneurology, psycholinguistics and psychophysiology and states that equipped with this knowledge 'the student should be ready to tackle the diagnostic study and teaching of children who find language learning difficult'. She emphasises the rigour of the undertaking and, indeed, it does take all her bright images to make it attractive. Fortunately, an alternative is offered. 'The student will find greater profit in studying the *profiles* of children who are handicapped by disabilities in language than by discursive chapters on symptoms and aetiology' (1969, p. 4). The emphasis on language profiles as a valuable way of understanding language disorders, has been a continuing feature for the last 20 years. All texts on the subject make use of a variety of case histories to indicate the range, diversity and also the common features of the condition.

By 1972, Leonard recommends the use of the term 'language impairment', in the context of a review that delineates research findings based around a *psycholinguistic model*, rather than considering 'aphasia' as a condition within a medical model. The end of that decade saw the widespread use of 'developmental language disorder', and 'developmental language impairment' as terms in clinical use, as well as in the research literature. Thus it was the confidence lent from considerations of language outside of a medical model that spurred the growth of interest in developmental language disorders as an area of research.

Table 1.2 shows profiles of two children with the terminology common to the 1960s and to the present day. These two profiles have been selected from the literature because they deal with very different children. There can therefore be no attempt to make direct comparison between them in order to suggest the improvement of one kind of terminology over another. The case described by Greene could be assessed and described today with only slight differences in terminology and an extended range of procedures. The case presented by Conti-Ramsden and Gunn would not have been described earlier within the language impairment category because speech and language therapists lacked the techniques and concepts to work with such children. Both cases (Greene, 1964; Conti-Ramsden and Gunn, 1986) should be read in full for the issues they raise and the insights they reveal.

A theoretical framework: models of language processing

Reliance upon case history study alone is unwise because no student can hope to encounter the whole range of language disorders thereby. It is necessary to have some kind of *theoretical framework* within which each individual aspect can be placed. It may fall to the psychologist or speech-language pathology researcher to generate a model that accounts for all the variables and allows them to be tested. The therapist

Table 1.2 Changes in terminology for assessment and classification

Assessment of Julie in 1964*		Assessment of Tony in 1986†	
Age at assessment (years)	4; 7	Age at assessment (years)	3; 4
Developmental history	Pneumonia at 9 months with anoxia and loss of consciousness Delayed milestones: walked at 18 months	Developmental history	General development normal Excellent self-help skills Early communication development normal Stopped communicating and responding to language in second year
Speech development	No babbling First words at 4 years Some difficulty with chewing and swallowing		
		Hearing	Within normal limits
Merrill–Palmer Scale	CA 4;6 MA 5;1	Assessment through observation	The following functions were described over time: pragmatic verbal comprehension syntax and phonology non-verbal abilities
Speech assessment	Could imitate individual consonants but had difficulty organising phonemic sequences No dyspraxia Poor auditory retention Unable to imitate even a simple rhythm No hearing loss Good auditory discrimination	Progress	There is progression from purely imitative responses to appropriate responses although some language forms presented difficulty Spontaneous conversation initiated at 5;4 years
		Standardized tests of language	Scored very poorly at 4 years RDLS CA 6;11 Age level 4;11 PLS CA 6;11 Age equiv. 6;6
Subsequent assessment measures	Terman-Merrill IQ 91 WISC CA 8:6 Verbal scale 86 Performance 93 Peabody CA 8;6 Peabody MA 6;1 Bender-Gestalt Performed poorly	Cognition	Consistently scored above average on Leiter International Performance Scale However, appeared to have specific non-verbal difficulties in areas of verbal reasoning distinguishing between essential/accidental information and developing generalised flexible scripts
Diagnosis	*Developmental aphasia* Difficulties in auditory recall and comprehension of abstract speech; impaired syntax and grammar	Diagnosis	*Semantic–pragmatic language disorder* Conversational disability

*From Greene (1964).
†From Conti-Ramsden and Gunn (1986).

and teacher will share the interest in constructing and testing such models. (For the latter the search for a common underlying cause may be of less interest than the search for a method that will allow many language-disordered children to be helped, but the relationship between therapy and empirical enquiry grows ever closer, as more speech and language therapists become established in research.)

It is difficult to handle all the possibilities of language impairment without some concept of how language is processed by the brain. The move away from looking at language disorders as a number of discrete entities makes it necessary to postulate a framework within which they can be seen as points on a continuum. The continuum will cover factors within the individual's ability to process language and those outside or environmental factors that impinge upon this processing. The severity of the disorder will also depend upon the profundity of the breakdown and the number of processes that are involved. Models of language processing will be discussed more fully in Chapter 4. They are also explored in a number of other texts; excellent discussions being offered by Butler (1984) and Harris and Coltheart (1986). They arise from theories of information processing as these can be focused upon language. Even a simple model of language processing must include the following stages

- Communicative intent and content to be communicated.
- A framework through which expression can be made.
- Assembly of a motor programme to execute the communication.
- Execution of the programme through organised sequences of neuro-muscular actions.
- Signal detection or awareness of stimulus.
- Attention to the stimulus also involving rejection of accompanying noise.
- Recognition.
- Memory
- Synthesis of all the above in order to build up a composite of all the information.

It is not difficult to consider such a model as it can be applied to the perfected skill. An adult well versed in communication makes use of all the above and has the ability to reflect upon their performance. Thus not only language but meta-language is involved. When the model is applied to the *development of language* it becomes more difficult to ascertain how routes through the model are established. Berger (1987) points out the difficulty of translating phenomena associated with the mature state to 'the realm of emerging forms and indefinite boundaries'. Some application can be made in that we may be able to identify points of breakdown or difficulty in the child's emerging skill. What is more taxing is to sort out the time when this difficulty heralds a permanent handicap or the point at which the child is unable to compensate by means of their other abilities.

Continuum of disability

Reference has already been made to a continuum of language disability. This implies that a language problem will continue to spread from its roots and pervade other aspects of development. It is this *pervasion of a number of skills* that makes the condition difficult to define and difficult to treat. In 1977 Strominger and Bashir presented a study based upon clinical records of language-disordered children first seen in the clinic at under 5 years of age and subsequently seen between the ages of 9 and 11. They reported that no child was entirely free from residual deficits. Examination of a number of aspects of language and learning showed a wide range of abnormality. The authors suggested that children who failed to acquire oral language would have difficulty in the acquisition of all language systems because of general problems posed by the grammar and its representation, regardless of form. Only 5% of the children in their sample had reading skills appropriate for their age. None of the children had been diagnosed as learning disabled and their educational failure was thus specifically linked to their language failure.

Byers Brown and Beveridge (1979) in an introduction to a workshop for teachers posed a number of questions representing queries that have recurred throughout the history of language disorders.

• Is there a continuum of language disturbances seen initially in the acquisition of the spoken word and later revealed as deficits in the secondary systems of reading and writing?

Most authorities incline to answer 'yes' (Aram and Nation, 1980; Wiig and Semel, 1984; King, Jones and Lasky, 1982; Cooper, 1985). Anecdotally and empirically (Silva, McGee and Williams, 1983; Bishop and Adams, 1990), the evidence points firmly to an ill-understood connection between early language deficits and later literacy skills.

• Can we assume that all children with initial disorders of language must be at risk educationally?

The answer to the second question is almost certainly 'yes' if we can also assume that the initial disorders were correctly diagnosed as affecting language and not articulation of speech. Where the child presents with initial problems of speech production only, pervasive language difficulty with its implications for education is not the likely outcome. Although Snowling (1987) proposes a link between the development of phonological coding skills and later reading failure, longitudinal research has shown that there is not necessarily a direct link. Bishop and Adams (1990) found that children whose phonological output deficits had resolved by age 5 were not at risk for reading failure. Those who were at risk for reading failure (and especially reading comprehension failure) were children presenting with persistent language deficits who had difficulty in synthesising a number of language processes.
• Is there one underlying factor that is causal and thereby links all

language manifestations? Or, are the skills all related by factors in the child's disposition, neurological, emotional or environmental but not causally linked?

- Are different language and learning problems occurring independently in vulnerable children rather than being bound together by one definable disability?

The answers to the last two questions are not readily available and the considerations which they require will be pursued in Chapters 2 and 7. Because Chapter 2 deals with identification, it will discuss those populations within which the language-disordered are most likely to be found as well as discussing their identifying signs. The discussion of clinical subtypes in Chapter 7 will consider how relationships between certain behaviour may be traced.

Differentiation

The process of differentiating language disorders has comprised three main approaches:

1. Attempts to differentiate between types of *abnormal language behaviour* occurring in a range of handicapping conditions.

The emergence of children who appeared to be deaf but failed to respond to methods of education designed for deaf or hearing-impaired children, led such pioneers as McGinnis in the USA and the Ewings in the UK to postulate the existence of aphasia in children as a separate entity and to try to find positive ways of identifying and treating it. The difficulty of making a positive identification is shown by cases of children who have had their diagnoses changed several times (Morley, 1973; Browning, 1987). A number of children had been shown to suffer from high frequency hearing loss in addition to developmental aphasia, which made diagnosis doubly difficult.

Major attention has long been focused upon children who show abnormal responses to sound because these have become associated with continuing difficulties in comprehending or processing spoken language. While the distinction between impaired auditory acuity and language disorder has become theoretically clear, it remains difficult to demonstrate in practice, particularly with extremely young children. Procedures for differential diagnosis are regularly revised and advocated (Ward and McCartney, 1978; Ward and Kellett, 1982; Ward, 1984).

The need to differentiate between those children who were generally delayed in all aspects of cognition and those who were language-disordered was stimulated by advances in both fields. The opening up of the whole field of learning difficulties in the last two decades has emphasised the importance of language in all aspects of teaching and training.

This has led to better methods of assessment of language potential. Advances in linguistic knowledge and the awareness of how language is used in intelligence testing has shown us more clearly how language-disordered children may be penalised by such tests. Differentiation between the two groups is being made possible by the development of progressively refined and sophisticated measures of intelligence. However, considerable caution is necessary still in interpreting such measures because of the complex relationship between cognitive and linguistic ability. To some extent, children's responses to sensitive teaching are an excellent guide to their overall intellectual ability. But if their language disorders are not recognised, the wrong demands may be placed upon them and their potential left unrealised (see also Chapter 8).

Differentiation between autism and language disorder, or more specifically the aphasic type of language disorder, has received the continuous attention of Rutter and his colleagues (Rutter, Bartak and Newman, 1971; Bartak, Rutter and Cox, 1975; Rutter, 1984; Rutter and Lord, 1987). Their investigations have illuminated both conditions. The distinction between the groups is a difficult one to make because of the frequency of overlapping symptoms. The type of language disorder most frequently associated with autism at the present time is that where the children show semantic–pragmatic difficulties. These are shown in the case studies of Conti-Ramsden and Gunn (1986), Byers Brown and Beveridge (1979), McTear (1985), and the group study of Bishop and Adams (1989). The quest for differentiation between the two groups owes as much to scholarly as to remedial demands because the conditions are still imperfectly understood.

2. Attempts to differentiate between the *rate and manner* in which language is normally acquired in infancy and abnormalities in this acquisition.

The slow emergence of linguistic features is a recognised characteristic of language disorder. Research and teaching efforts during the last decade have enabled us to document these features much more accurately than was previously possible. Conspicuous in this field is the work of Crystal who, together with colleagues, pioneered and propagated linguistic profiling (Crystal, Fletcher and Garman, 1976; Crystal, 1982b). This has many advantages over previous methods of representing the child's language level because it identifies the imbalances or mismatches between linguistic systems. It is consequently possible to distinguish at an early age between overall delay affecting all aspects of language and specific delays affecting one or more systems, at least with respect to the formal aspects of language.

Menyuk in the USA was one of the first to draw attention to the importance of documenting the rate of linguistic feature acquisition and her early work on phonology has been followed by the major studies of Ingram in the USA (1974, 1976, 1987) and Grunwell in the UK (1975, 1980b, 1981). At the same time, interest was developing in measuring the other components of language, namely grammatical structure, vocabulary acquisition and use, and functional or interpersonal use of language. The last item was temporarily submerged in the 1960s and 1970s whilst more exact structural measurements were being pursued. It was brought into prominence in the UK through the work of Halliday (1975) and also through the studies of the American psychologist Bruner (1983a, b). The attention this functional or pragmatic aspect of language has subsequently received has more than made amends for any temporary neglect (McTear and Conti-Ramsden, 1992). It has been greatly stimulated by research into infant behaviour and mother–child interaction.

Writers in the 1970s were considerably occupied with the distinction between delayed and deviant development of spoken language. Byers Brown (1976) expressed one view in the following way (it was previously pointed out that 'speech' is here synonymous with 'spoken language'):

> Delayed speech involves the late appearance of words and their combination into phrases and sentences. Rudimentary utterance and general behaviour may be on normal lines but the speech is less mature and less accomplished than is considered appropriate for the child's age or common among his peers. The utterance would be suitable to a younger child and could be found in the normal developmental sequence. The delay may also be apparent in the child's phonology or in his use of speech to control his environment.
>
> Deviant speech does not fit into a normal developmental sequence. It may manifest itself in voice or tone quality, sound structure or sound sequence. While gross deviations are likely to be associated with pathology, deviant phonological or syntactical constructions can occur in the absence of pathology, suggesting that the child is having difficulty in making deductions from the stream of sounds he hears or that he is not able to make use of his deductions to build up his language system in a conventional manner.

These conclusions were based upon the study of a clinical population considered retrospectively. They were not necessarily shared by investigators conducting research across large groups of language-delayed children. Some investigators considered that the term 'deviant' was never appropriate to developing language, which contained phonemes and other linguistic structures that were normally produced but which occurred late or in unusual combination. [For further discussion of the use of 'delayed' and 'deviant' language, see Menyuk and Looney (1972) and Leonard (1972).] Byers Brown's description of 'delayed speech' might be subsumed under 'immature' or 'transient' delays and her 'deviant speech' under 'true delay leading to disorder'. We appear to circle around the position that there is a group of children whose speech appears late or emerges slowly but which improves spontaneously and another group sharing the same broad characteristics but which does not improve. We know a great deal more about the large heterogeneous group that does not improve but we remain in the frustrating position of being able to identify both groups only in retrospect, i.e. when improvement has or has not taken place. Another factor that is much better considered now is the possible extent of normal variation within language acquisition. We are now aware that although normal children master the same language skills they may adopt different strategies in order to do so (Shore, 1995). The more we know about these different strategies, the more we must question a simple division into normal and abnormal language acquisition.

Current consensus indicates that the preoccupations of previous researchers with the form of language and its deviance should now be put aside in favour of more productive debates. There is now overwhelming evidence to suggest that the syntactic output of language-impaired children is rarely deviant and that the order of acquisition of language structures follows that of the normal child, but at a much slower rate (Curtiss, Katz and Tallal, 1992). That is not to say that the language-disordered child always sounds like a younger child. A subjective impression of deviance in language usually arises from an interaction of factors from various domains of language or a mismatch between levels of language development. For instance, a child with a word-finding deficit may struggle with retrieval of lexical items to the extent that there is rarely a complete sentence in his verbal output. Another child may have adequate syntactic skills, but impoverished development of the use of language, so that his ability to communicate ideas is out of step with his formal language ability. We can only afford to reject totally the notion of disorder or deviancy (as opposed to delay) if we take a narrow view of language as a syntactic enterprise.

3. Attempts to differentiate between types of developmental language disorder.

The first differentiation between subgroups of conditions in which language failed to emerge normally was between receptive and expressive conditions. Each of these was then examined for further distinctions. One of the first attempts at subtype differentiation by a British speech and language therapist was that of Greene (1963). Taking the broadly expressive group of disorders, Greene described one set of children whose delayed speech was associated with coordination disorder and another where there was language learning difficulty. Cooper and Griffiths (1978) subsequently presented a broad classification drawn from a sample of several hundred 6-year-old children with 'developmental dysphasia'. This was to be seen as a simple classification based upon the way the children presented in the classroom. All the children were free from major mental or physical handicaps. The classification contains five categories:

- Children who demonstrate normal hearing upon audiometry but who show little or no ability to comprehend or use speech.
- Children with varying degrees of hearing loss who have failed to respond to the use of sound amplification and the normal methods of teaching the deaf in that they have not acquired comprehension or use of spoken language.
- Children with normal or near normal comprehension but with absence or severe retardation of spoken language.
- A similar group to the above but one in which spoken language shows a late onset (3–4 years) and then develops rapidly with only residual traces of difficulty at 7–8 years. However, these children show severe reading difficulties.
- Children who develop a grasp of the mechanics of speech but whose use is often imitative, stereotyped and irrelevant.

In this relatively early classification system, there is a recognition of the complex nature of language disorders and the diversity of the conditions with which the clinician is faced. Further attempts at differentiation followed are described more fully in Chapter 5. The authors describe each category fully in their text. Readers may judge for themselves the amount of progress in classification that has been made since Cooper and Griffiths' paper. Despite repeated attempts at differentiation at this level, it should be noted that the refinement of categories within the population does not necessarily teach us more about the range and extent of the disorder although it appears to be an advance on individual clinical observation.

Conclusion

The identification of the child with a developmental language disorder is still sometimes a taxing procedure, even for the experienced speech-language clinician. The difficulties of clinical identification seem almost an echo of the years of research and clinical reporting that has been assimilated to establish a notion of developmental language disorder. Once a problem has been identified, the way is cleared for further elaboration of its characteristics, and it is to this process that we will now turn.

Chapter 2
Identification

Summary

This chapter surveys the way in which language disorder can be identified. It considers some of the ideas that have been presented on both causal and associated factors with emphasis upon the part these play in identification. The multifactorial nature of language disorder is illustrated and the identification process is discussed. Early screening methods are examined and some evaluation made as to their merits and disadvantages. Particular attention is paid to the factors that must be considered when trying to predict language disorders from early language delay.

How can these children be found?

The prevailing philosophy of therapeutic intervention is that it should start as early as possible. There are many humane arguments to be used in support. The earlier a child is helped to come to terms with his disability, the more likely he is to find ways in which to help himself. The earlier the parents are given help and support, the more likely is the whole family to behave positively and hopefully. The earlier that education authorities are informed as to potential needs for special provision, the more chance there is of that provision being available. The sooner acquainted everyone in the child's environment is with his abilities and his needs, the easier it will be for him to receive encouragement and acceptance. The validity of these arguments, together with the economic factors upon which they impinge, will be discussed more thoroughly in Chapter 7. If they have any validity at all, however, then early identification, which logically precedes intervention, must take place as soon as possible.

There are also academic arguments to support the need for early identification. The sooner a condition is properly noted and described the better will be the chances of tracking its course. This will increase understanding. It has not been easy for past investigators to distinguish between the effects of the underlying condition itself and those effects

23

which come about as the child tries to help or to protect himself from failure. The withdrawal, aggression and hyperactivity that some children show are only three of the behaviours that can make approach more difficult. There are many aspects of the children's behaviour that can compound their difficulties either through disguising the basic deficiency or by antagonising those who try to help them. If we are to understand how language disorders develop, we need to know how they start.

It has been pointed out (Byers Brown, 1987) that our ideas as to what constitutes early identification are under constant revision as our knowledge accrues. Two decades ago we would have been thinking about the 3-year-old. Now our interest in emergent language and our greatly increased knowledge in all aspects of child development make us look for signs of abnormality during the period when normal language is acquired, i.e. the first 3 years of life. We also know more about the factors that place a child at risk for developmental disorders in the biological sense and of those environmental and social circumstances that compound the risk. We may therefore start to identify developmental language disorders by looking at the settings in which they are most likely to be found.

It would be misleading to suggest that language disorders are only identified in infancy or early childhood. The identification may be made by the class teacher who realises that the difficulty a pupil is having in learning to read is outside the range of normal variation, or in later years is falling behind peers in language work. Identification may come about through a social worker who perceives antisocial behaviour in an adolescent as stemming from basic communication problems. We cannot hope to identify all developmental language disorders at the time when the bases of language are being laid down even though this must be our aim. So all parents and professionals must be encouraged to understand how the disorders may manifest themselves. This aspect of public education will be considered more thoroughly in the next chapter.

What do we know about these children?

Family history

The first textbook devoted to genetic aspects of speech and language disorders was published in 1983 (Ludlow and Cooper, 1983), and subsequently several researchers have investigated the familial background of children with language impairment, in the quest to ascertain the true nature of developmental language disorders. Whereas it is suspiciously obvious that this should be one of the primary areas of research for those searching for a 'cause', there are two major pitfalls in this field. Firstly, to show convincingly that there is a familial factor in language

impairment is important, but it does not tell us any more about management than we already knew, save that the disorder is not only due to
environmental influences. Rather we must take the broader view that the
studies referred to in this section contribute to a body of theoretical
knowledge, which will ultimately advance the field. Secondly, and more
immediately, it is imperative to be critical about such research. The
major projects investigating genetic influences have been altruistic in
their aims, but have, crucially, drawn from subtly different populations,
and this results in difficulties of comparison between and across studies.

Edwards quotes from the findings of a multi-centre study (Edwards et
al., 1984) involving 187 children with ages from 3 to 6 years. These children were referred from the regular clinic clientele of participating therapists with a diagnosis of 'language disorder' and no other significant
handicaps. Of the 187 children, 55% of the boys and 39% of the girls had
blood relatives with some kind of speech disability. This figure prompted
the authors to speculate that, if a genetic factor is involved, boys are
more vulnerable.

Both Robinson (1987) and Sonksen (1979) found risk factors in
familial conditions to be higher in boys than in girls. The highest risk is
for brothers of boys and the lowest for sisters of girls. Robinson studied
the records of children from Moor House School, a residential school for
children with severe disorders of speech and language. From this population, he quotes a total figure of 40% for children with some positive
family history, 28% having a parent or sibling. Haynes and Naidoo
(1991), taking a group of children from a special school in England,
found 53.8% of these children to have at least one relative with a history
of speech or language difficulty, or 41% within the nuclear family. The
presumption is that there is a genetic factor operating in both severe and
moderate language disorders but as yet, aetiology with a single locus has
not been revealed. The fact that even though siblings may show language
disorders they are not necessarily as severe as those shown by the target
child, is only one indication of the complex nature of the aetiology.

These findings have been updated by rigorous research on both sides
of the Atlantic. In the USA, Tallal, Ross and Curtiss (1989), by gathering
data from parents by questionnaire regarding 76 language-impaired and
54 normal children, found that both mothers and fathers of experimental subjects were more likely to report a history of speech/language
or other educational difficulty than were the control subjects' parents.
There was also a higher rate of affected siblings reported. Similarly,
Tomblin (1989) and Tomblin and Buckwalter (1994) found evidence for
the concentration of language problems within families. Their research
and that of others (Tallal et al., 1991) has also crucially shown that the
genotype (the genetic profile) of the individuals with SLI whom they
studied, although present, did not always necessarily lead to frank
language disorder. That is, despite having the genetic predisposition for

language impairment, these children did not reliably show the language features of SLI. Such 'incomplete penetrance' (Tomblin and Buckwalter, 1994) suggests that other factors may be involved in the development of an impaired language system, a conclusion that Bishop (1992a) had come to from a different route (see below).

Both Tallal et al. (1991) and Tomblin were studying a heterogeneous group of children defined as language-impaired. Would the picture be any different if subject selection were more closely constrained? The studies coordinated by Whitehurst (Whitehurst et al., 1988, 1991), focused on children with *expressive language delay* and no evidence was found for a familial factor. This was at odds with most other family surveys (for example, Lahey and Edwards, 1995). It is important to note that Whitehurst et al. felt that there could be a different finding if other groups had been under consideration (see also Whitehurst and Fischel, 1994). Specifically, they argued that the nature of expressive language delay and expressive–receptive delays were different, and that one might anticipate different results were the latter group to have been included. Future studies might clarify these issues by careful delineation of group characteristics, but the numbers of subjects needed and the difficulties imposed by recruitment bias make these very difficult studies to pursue.

Another option is to study the pedigree of a single family, and whereas such findings are of restricted theoretical interest, they provide evidence that at least some language disorders can be attributed to genetic factors. An example of this sort of study is that of Gopnik and Crago (1991) who plotted out the pedigree of a family who, interestingly enough, presented with severe expressive language difficulties. The family had 16 out of 30 members affected by similar phonological/grammatical problems across three generations. This study is of especial importance because it shows, fairly convincingly, that it is possible not to just inherit a language disorder, but to inherit the same *type* of language disorder. The precise genetic mechanism operating within the Gopnik and Crago family is suspected to be a single, autosomally dominant gene (Crago and Gopnik, 1994). It has to be pointed out that the type of language disorder in this family was unusually true to type through the generations, and that many other types of language impairment may not lend themselves so well to phenotyping. Such studies, however, together with increasingly sophisticated genetic marking techniques, point the way to the future (see also Lewis, 1990; Pembrey, 1992).

In the UK, Haynes and Naidoo (1991) found that there was a slightly higher rate of positive family history in their 'Classic' group (see Chapter 5), but this finding was non-significant. Bishop (1992a) examined the speech and language of 61 pairs of twins. Twin studies have much to tell us about the genetic influences on a wide variety of conditions and have been used in the past by a number of researchers into autism, stuttering, etc. As Bishop points out, there is a need to proceed to this level of investigation if one is seriously interested in the nature of the disorder. Familial incidences are useful, but clouded by numerous other environmental factors affecting a family through generations. Bishop's twins had determined zygosity, a non-verbal IQ of 85 or over and a history of present or past specific language impairment. The finding of a very high rate of language disorder in co-twins of an affected child reinforces the notion of SLI as an inherited disorder. Bishop also found some evidence for greater similarity in the type of language impairment in monozygotic rather than dizygotic twins. Similar results are reported by Lewis and Thompson (1992) in their twin study, which was based on parental report rather than direct testing as in the Bishop study. Lewis and Thompson conclude that the genetic factors underlying the articulatory apparatus and cognitive systems may account for the higher degree of concordance in monozygotic twins affected.

The evidence of familial incidence of developmental disorder may help identification in a broad epidemiological sense but cannot necessarily be expected to pick up the individual child. We cannot assume that all parents will react with prompt concern to early signs of disordered language because they have experienced difficulties themselves or in other offspring. Whilst it is likely that memories of their own distress will prompt them to seek help for their child earlier rather than later, it is also possible that the condition will cause less than usual concern because it is familiar. Parents' attitudes and beliefs will affect their behaviour quite as much as will their knowledge. Research into family histories will help to identify the individuals who are most at risk but it is not likely to prevent the births of more at-risk infants. Although the penalties for language disorder can be very high, they are not the kind of penalties that prevent people from having children.

Chromosomal abnormalities

The preceding paragraph does not necessarily apply in those cases where language impairment is part of a syndrome giving rise to other major handicaps (e.g. Duchenne-type muscular dystrophy). Such conditions do not account for any substantial proportion of language disorders and neither do the chromosomal abnormalities that have been found in association with grossly delayed expressive speech. Garvey and Mutton selected nine children from a pool of 450 with severe speech and language problems. These nine children had normal comprehension for speech but grossly delayed expression. The children thus constituted a special subtype. Of the nine cases studied, three showed chromosomal abnormalities (Garvey and Mutton, 1973). Robinson (1987) gives a figure of 3–5% of all children with developmental language disorders as having some kind of chromosomal abnormalities. This figure is based upon several different studies. Follow-up studies of infants found on new-born screening to have chromosomal abnormalities, reveal that about half of these infants show delay in language development or show speech problems. Robinson, again basing his deductions on the results of a number of studies, says that the communication problems are most consistently demonstrated in boys with Klinefelter's syndrome but are also seen in XYY boys. However, not all children with these chromosomal abnormalities show delayed language development nor is it always severe and persistent in those who do so. The Fragile-X chromosome syndrome has been associated with delayed language development although the relationship between the two has yet to be thoroughly explored. Wolf-Schein et al. (1987) have presented data to argue that the language impairment in Fragile-X syndrome cannot be entirely explained by the level of learning difficulties. In the Haynes and Naidoo study, which looked solely at children with specific speech and language difficulties, a significant number of subjects (15%) were found to have chromosomal abnormalities of various kinds (though the numbers of children involved were small).

A medically-based aetiology

The search for one main causative factor that can be revealed through medical examination has not been productive. The consensus of opinion is that there is no one overriding aetiology. Nevertheless there are factors that medical examination cannot overlook because they have been shown to be associated with delayed or abnormal language development. Careful examination must be made to exclude the two main causes of language delay in children, namely hearing loss and general intellectual impairment. The most common factor between language disorders that is not associated with these two groups is some degree of neurological impairment. Language disorders have been shown to coexist with mild types of cerebral palsy and with clumsiness. It is reasonable to look towards a damaged nervous system to unite the many different perceptual–motor problems that are encountered in the language-disordered population. The possible roles of brain abnormalities and brain damage are discussed by Goodman (1987). He observes that: 'At present, the hypothesis that all developmental language disorders have a neurological basis is attractive but unproven'.

Neurological explanations of developmental language disorder

Goodman states that neurological explanations tend to fall into one of three groups: maturational lag, atypical lateralisation and focal abnormality.

Maturational lag

The theory of maturational lag is appealing to many because, as Goodman points out: 'Everyday experience teaches us that children mature at different rates and that the same child may mature quickly in one area and slowly in another'. Rutter (1984), in propounding the theory, suggests that 'unusually great variations in rates of brain maturation might be responsible for specific delays in the development of particular brain functions (such as speech or language)' (p. 584). The support for maturational lag as a general aetiology for language disorders is weak but authors indicate that it could account for some of them. The theory would be expected to account for those children who show early delays in language development but who eventually catch up with their peers. Stark, Mellits and Tallal (1983) discuss this group of language-delayed children and contrast them with a group considered to be severely language-impaired. The language-impaired children are likely to present a number of deficits in perceptual and motor skills or a few very severe deficits. These deficits, together with the language impairment and possible difficulty in interacting with other people, could be associated with significant neurological impairment. The authors do not state the possible neurological association with language delay. They suggest that some of the skills underpinning language may not emerge sufficiently to contribute to the child's language learning at the usual time. Consequently there may be temporary but marked delay in that aspect of language. As the child perceives the nature and use of language more clearly, and as other aspects of the whole process appear, there may be acceleration of language development.

Bishop and Edmundson (1987a) have considered the distinction between the two groups made by Stark, Mellits and Tallal (1983) in the light of their own research findings. This consideration prompted them to test out the hypothesis of maturational lag as it might apply to a language-delayed and a language-impaired group. They suggested that if the language-delayed children developed at a normal rate after a slow start, maintaining the same intervals between language milestones, the children 'would be aptly described as having maturational lag' (Bishop and Edmundson, 1987b). The language-impaired children should be characterised by slow rates of development with verbal skills plateauing early. Thus the theoretical position could be tested by testing the prediction that the rate of language development would be different between the groups. A second approach was to look for evidence of immaturity in the motor functioning of the language-delayed group. The authors cite Wolff, Gunnoe and Cohen (1985) that neuromotor measures provide reliable criteria for developmental age in young children. If the language-delayed children showed initial immaturity of neuromotor function with gradual improvement, it would be evidence of overall maturation. The language-impaired children would not be expected to show this improvement because they were considered to have more significant neuropathology. Bishop and Edmundson failed to find differentiating factors between the two groups on the lines anticipated. There was no distinctive difference in the rate of progress made by the children when assessed at intervals by a verbal test battery. Nor was it possible to differentiate between the groups on the grounds of simple motor maturation. The investigators concluded that both subgroups seemed to be best accounted for in terms of brain maturation because both groups made steady progress after a delayed start. They note problems that challenge the maturational lag hypothesis as a general aetiology, however. These concern the uneven pattern of language impairment that is not indicative of immaturity; also the logical fact that if maturational lag rather than neurological impairment is present, children should eventually catch up rather than show persisting problems in a number of language and language-related skills.

Locke (1994) proposed that language unfolds in the child in a fixed sequence of stages. The basis of language impairment, as he sees it, is a genetically determined slow maturation of species-specific neural mechanisms, which leads to an under elaboration of linguistic knowledge, with a consequent failure to activate the analytic mechanisms necessary for the further acquisition of language. The result of this, states Locke, will be exactly what we find; a child with a specific language problem and a family history of language impairment. The investigation of language delay from a neuro-scientific viewpoint may provide greater insight into the processes involved.

Atypical lateralisation

The literature on cerebral lateralisation in relation to disorders of language and fluency is considerable and controversial. Even if the coexistence of some of the phenomena were proven, it is not possible to tease out cause and effect. Empirical evidence suggests that laterality, as demonstrated in handedness studies may not be a factor in early language delay (Bishop 1990; Whitehurst and Fischel, 1994). Even Haynes and Naidoo (1991), testing very impaired children, could find no conclusive evidence of abnormal laterality in the majority of cases.

Focal abnormalities

Focal abnormalities have been cited as a possible cause for the failure of development of particular skills, but even with modern imaging techniques still 'little is known of the neuropathology of developmental language disorders' (Robinson, 1991). Plante et al. (1991) and Plante (1991) have initiated the search for brain abnormalities from imaging techniques. Boys with specific language impairment, as well as some of their siblings and parents were shown to have atypical perisylvian asymmetries. These asymmetries are thought to have arisen in utero as the result of genetic influences. Researchers have not been able to demonstrate convincingly the presence of focal lesions as explanations of developmental language impairment. Even if neurological factors are not responsible for all cases of disordered language in developing children, they appear sufficiently frequently to make all infants at risk for abnormal neurological development also at risk for abnormal language development.

Perinatal factors

One population of infants that is held to be at risk for neurological impairment is the premature or pre-term population and particularly babies of very low birth weight. These babies should therefore be followed up at regular intervals to see that their language, among other skills, is developing normally. Evidence to date has been contradictory. Stevenson, Bax and Stevenson (1982) found no statistically significant association between either the gestational age of the child or the birth weight and speech and language delay at the age of 3, although there was a non-significant trend in the expected direction. Bax (1987) considers that the relationship is still unclear and reminds us that because both low birth weight and speech and language delay are common in most developed countries, chance associations will occur.

Wright et al. (1983) found a significant difference between the language status of low birth weight and normal infants when assessed at 3;5 years. Byers Brown, Bendersky and Chapman (1986) also found a significant delay in the development of the speech–sound system in preterm infants as compared with the normal population. The trend was more marked in infants who had sustained intraventricular haemorrhage (IVH), the range of delay being wider. On the other hand, Menyuk, Liebergott and Schultz (1986) found no significant differences in the lexical or phonological development of premature and full-term infants when measures were taken at intervals during the second and third years of life, and in a subsequent phase of their study (Menyuk et al., 1991), found that premature infants were within normal limits on a range of linguistic and cognitive tests. Aram et al. (1991) addressed the issue of the presence of specific language impairment, as opposed to language lag, in very low birth-weight children. Their findings reveal no significantly different rate of specific language impairment in the premature group as compared with controls, but there was evidence of an increased rate of language delay associated with other developmental problems in the low birth-weight group.

The above findings turn out to be less contradictory when all of the associated variables have been examined. Wright et al. (1983) emphasise the importance of social and environmental factors in influencing language development and thus helping infants to achieve normal language levels in their preschool years despite the initial effects of prematurity. Byers Brown, Bendersky and Chapman (1986) express considerable caution about the predictive value of their findings. In fact, subsequent research (Lewis and Bendersky, 1989) has shown that the number of medical complications correlated most highly with language skill whether or not IVH had occurred. The authors suggest that development of the preterm child be studied with an interactional view of various factors such as medical complications and socio-economic status, which could have an impact upon each other. The relationship between environmental factors and speech and language development had not been adequately established with regard to perinatal conditions. In order to assess the importance of any one factor, such as prematurity, the possible influence of many circumstances that are associated with it (single parents' status, poverty, malnutrition) have to be teased out and separately considered as by Lewis and Bendersky. There is still scope for further investigation along the lines that Bishop has implied (1992a): that developmental language disorders may be the result of interaction of genetic, perinatal, and possibly other environmental factors.

It will be apparent from the discussion so far that whilst certain medical and environmental factors may place children at risk for language disorder, they do not, in themselves, identify them. Language disorders can only be identified as language emerges or fails to emerge. Moreover, at the emergent stage there is no guarantee that the signs will be stable. Byers Brown (1987) quotes from a follow-up investigation of one of the IVH children in the 1986 study. When first assessed, the child was 16 months of age or 13 months corrected age. Findings were as follows:

Bayley Scales of Mental and Motor Development	Mental scale	69
	Motor scale	99
Sequenced Inventory of Communication Development	Receptive age	8 months
	Expressive age	12 months
Speech–sound estimate		9 months

The picture appeared to be one of cognitive and linguistic delay with strengths on the motor side. However, when reassessed at the age of 3;4 years, the balance had shifted:

Stanford Binet Intelligence Scales	Test composite	95
Sequenced Inventory of Communicative Ability	Receptive age	36 months
	Expressive age	36 months

The mean length of utterance (MLU) calculated from a spontaneous speech sample gave an age equivalent of 35 months. This child would no longer be considered as language or cognitively delayed. Although on the low side of average, he is not significantly retarded. At the same time he is recorded as showing some movement disorder and his speech is not easily intelligible due to immature articulation. At this age he appears to show greater difficulty with motor than with other skills. His case illustrates the caution that must be shown in predicting the course of language development in very young, damaged infants. The capacity of the nervous system to recover from insult sustained at an early age must be taken into account.

Other causal correlates

Otitis media

Otitis media became a prime contender for the role of chief causal agent in developmental language disorders as we moved into the 1980s. It had been demonstrated as early as 1970 (Owrid, 1970; Hamilton and Owrid, 1974) that the conductive hearing loss resulting from otitis media depressed verbal skills and educational attainments in school children. During the following decade attention became focused upon the effects of recurrent episodes of otitis media on the child's developing linguistic system. Anxiety was not only generated by evidence of sustained conductive loss but by the number of early episodes of otitis media suffered by the child. The broad questions posed were:

* Does otitis media lead to language disorder?
* Does otitis media always lead to conductive loss and thence to language delay?

Because otitis media is episodic and associated with fluctuations in hearing, children who encountered a number of episodes during their early development were deemed to be at particular risk in the acquisition of phonology and syntax. Fluctuating hearing losses in the region of 40 dB would mean that the infant failed to hear a number of important auditory/linguistic clues (e.g. tense, plurality). By causing confusion because of its fluctuations, the condition would prevent the acquisition of good listening skills that might allow the child to compensate. However, the otitis media argument was not just based upon the possible relationship between fluctuations in hearing and delays in mastering language structure.

In the USA, deductions were made from the results of animal experiments and these were then transferred to the human infant. Experimental studies using animals showed that deprivation of auditory stimulation could lead to atrophy of auditory function. It was then hypothesised that the effect of otitis media in infancy might be such as to cause recurrent conductive loss with consequent failure of the function of hearing to develop. This failure of development could not be compensated for by subsequent restoration to health of the middle ear. This theory was effectively challenged by Ventry (1980) and was subsequently replaced by studies that were most immediately related to the practical effects of conductive loss during the period of language learning. There have been a number of reviews of the role of otitis media as a long-term influence upon language development (Paradise, 1981; Bishop and Edmundson, 1986; Hasenstab, 1987) and a very large number of studies exploring the relationship (Jerger et al., 1983; Shriberg and Smith, 1983; Teele et al., 1984).

Attention has been directed to both comprehension and production of the language system and on both disorders and delays. Because the comprehension of spoken language depends upon the ability to hear a number of unstressed syllables and low energy, low volume sounds, it is logical to deduce that a fluctuating hearing loss that reduced this ability could be responsible for both delay and disorder. Because the ability to generate a sound system depends on knowledge of the sounds that are required by that system, it is also logical to attribute system failure to faulty information based upon hearing impairment. However, studies such as Bishop and Edmundson (1986), Roberts et al. (1991) and Gravel and Wallace (1992) failed to reveal a relationship between otitis media in early life and later language delay. Lonigan et al. (1992) did find a link between preschool expressive language delay and early episodes of otitis media. Their subjects later made rapid progress towards normal language levels. It is the data from such group studies that led Whitehurst and Fischel (1994) to conclude that 'otitis media does not seem to be a factor in the language progress of children whose language delays persist until four years of age'. This conclusion needs confirmation, according to Roberts and Schuele (1991) by prospective studies of infants with otitis media, carefully followed throughout their development, with accurate documentation of illness episodes and language performance.

Practising clinicians are as likely to be swayed in their judgements of the effects of otitis media by the children they treat as they are by research studies. Most speech and language therapists working with young children can cite instances where periods of conductive loss interfered markedly with a child's language learning. As speech and language therapists do not see children with otitis media, conductive loss and normal speech, they are not in a position to make judicial statements as to the importance of otitis media as a causal factor. Byers Brown (1981) cites the cases of three male children seen in the clinic during their fourth year of age (these are summarised in Table 2.1) . Each boy showed evidence of conductive hearing loss. In the first case, the diagnosis was of delayed speech and language and this was resolved within months of medical treatment that restored hearing to the normal level. In the second case the diagnosis of delayed language was complicated by hyperactivity and attentional problems leaving the role of conductive loss unclear. In fact, restoration of normal middle ear function was not followed by language improvement but by echolalia, continuing attentional difficulties and general linguistic immaturity. This would appear to be a case where the language disorder was primary and the hearing loss compounding.

The third child showing conductive hearing loss was also diagnosed as having a general developmental delay. However, good cognitive ability was revealed both through assessment and through observation and parental report. Speech was severely retarded. Treatment to alleviate the conductive hearing loss again restored middle ear function. There was no immediate increase in spoken language but progress in that area was steady and sustained. Verbal comprehension was within normal for age limits by the end of 6 months and verbal expression within a year. In this case, the hearing loss was also considered to be a compounding rather than a causal factor. The delayed language development was probably consequent upon maturational lag affecting a number of skills.

Individual case histories of this kind cannot be expected to resolve the broad questions posed at the start of this section. What they can do is to remind us of the need to explore the child's hearing levels and auditory behaviour before and during any treatment for delayed language. The significance of a conductive loss in relation to language development will vary according to the child's other abilities and deficits. Most investigators are convinced of the multifactorial nature of language disorders. While results of many of the investigations of otitis media and language disorder are inconclusive, few would be prepared to discount the possible adverse effects when combined with other predisposing factors. The weight of statistical evidence emerging from any forthcoming study of the relationship between otitis media, conductive hearing loss and language disorder should not interfere with the scrupulous appraisal of this relationship in any one child.

Cognitive impairment

The relationship between cognitive and language development is of major interest in attempting to specify the presence and the nature of a language disorder. The emergence of a child's first words has always been held to reveal his ability to think. First words are therefore a source of gratification and relief to parents and of particular interest to psychologists. Children who show delay in the onset of words and particularly word combinations may also show difficulties in verbal comprehension. Such children are likely to be at risk for general cognitive impairment particularly if they also show delay in the acquisition of motor skills. The more a child's delay is focused upon one aspect of

Table 2.1 Otitis media and developmental language disorder

Child	Age (years)	Presenting symptom	Hearing	Speech–language	Treatment	Outcome
Child A	3;8	Delayed speech	a/c loss 40–45 dB R 45 dB L b/c 5–10 dB Speech discrimination: Kendall Toy Test 50/55 dB Impedance showed poor compliance with negative middle ear pressures of −250 mmHg	Immature phonology and syntax Hyponasal voice quality	Adenoidectomy Myringotomy Language stimulation with focus on listening; auditory discrimination; vocabulary sentence expansion	Normal hearing Age appropriate syntax Resolving phonological immaturities Normal voice quality
Child B	3;3	Delayed speech Temper tantrums, hyperactivity	Variable responses to sounds but mainly 55–60 dB Would not allow impedance testing; subsequent otological examination revealed fluid	Immaturity in all aspects of language plus attention difficulty	Adenoidectomy and myringotomy Language stimulation plus attention control	Auditory behaviour still variable; broad scatter of responses to language assessment suggestive of primary language disorder
Child C	3;9	Delayed speech and delayed motor development	a/c 50 dB R and L b/c normal Impedance curves very flat with poor compliance and negative pressure	Severe retardation of expressive language with good comprehension	Tonsilectomy, adenoidectomy and myringotomy Language therapy with focus upon imitation, sound production discrimination, modelling and sentence expansion	Normal hearing Continued language therapy with emphasis on syntax until 5;0 years when performance was age appropriate

linguistic development, the more likely he/she is to be heading for a language, rather than a general intellectual, problem. However, this is to make only the broadest and simplest statement about the relationship. Language disorders may be so pervasive that they affect the developing child's ability to acquire verbal symbols and insightful language strategies. As a consequence his/her ability to demonstrate normal thought processes will be affected.

There is a very considerable body of work devoted to the development of both cognition and language and to their relative dependence or independence. The influence of this literature has been felt in both the diagnoses and remediation of language handicap. Early diagnoses tended to rest upon the discrepancy between verbal and non-verbal skills as demonstrated by intelligence tests. As the child grew older, tests became more heavily loaded verbally. So children who had been thought to be 'within normal limits' intellectually were found to show relatively low overall functioning in relation to their peers. Many questions arose from such results. The tests themselves were subjected to stringent criticism, the nature of language in problem solving was examined, and the performance of language-disordered children on a large number of cognitive processing tasks was explored.

Rice (1983), indicates the bewildering array of studies through which language-disordered children were found to perform more poorly than their peers with normal language and refers to a detectable sense of frustration regarding the elusiveness of cognition and its role in language impairment and of the remediation process. This kind of frustration was suffered by those in research more than by those in therapy where the interest and stimulation from cognitive exploration was very positive in its effects. The main focus was upon the very young child. Language therapists grasped the idea of early symbolic function as a vital precursor to language function. If symbolic activity was present in one domain, e.g. play, it not only indicated the potential for cognitive development but the possibility of transfer to another domain, that of verbal symbols. Play became a highly important diagnostic and therapeutic tool in the preschool language clinic. While the benefits were considerable in many associated areas, mother–child interaction, concentration and general well being, there was little research from the clinical side to affirm the transfer from one form of symbolic activity to another. Largo and Howard (1979) point out that the relationship between play behaviour and language acquisition has turned out to be more complex than at first supposed. Thal and Bates (1988) have offered evidence in support of a local homology whereby specific impairments in play may predict specific patterns of early language impairment. But the relationship between symbolic play, functional play and language development is still not clearly understood. There seems to be evidence for early correspondences (certainly in the one-word stage, Omura, 1991), but beyond that play and language seem to develop in parallel, rather than from a common base, and as Doswell et al.'s research suggests 'development may occur unevenly rather than always in parallel across the two domains' (Doswell et al., 1994).

Rice's paper explores the territory of linguistic and non-linguistic knowledge in relation to cognition. She shows that although each has its own domain, there is a sizeable area of overlap in which linkage is possible. The question of major interest is whether the language disordered experience most difficulty in the shared domain or in the territory peculiar to language. Benton (1978) in an earlier review looks at some of the evidence to support the view that dysphasia is the particular expression of a cognitive impairment affecting non-verbal as well as verbal behaviour. One such hypothesis deals with the processing of auditory information. This is a 'modal-specific' cognitive deficit and is indeed dealt with in the same volume (Tallal and Piercy, 1978) as a defect of auditory perception. We see here some of the difficulties confronting those who tried to separate auditory processing from other cognitive activities. Tests to demonstrate auditory processing difficulty could only be carried out with children who had achieved a fairly high level of cognitive function. Such testing therefore becomes specific cognitive testing and the hypothesis of an auditory sequencing impairment constituting the common denominator in language disorder cannot be upheld or refuted (for further discussion see Rees, 1973).

Generally speaking, the education of speech and language therapists has not equipped them for the cognitive exploration of language disorders that is now required. The present interest in pragmatic skills stimulates the need to find out how children become aware of other people in all sorts of contexts. Such awareness is known to be lacking in the language-disordered. We have to ascertain the extent to which this lack of insight is the product of unrealistic teaching and therapy and how much is part of the language disability. There are many other aspects to be examined. For example Lloyd (1982) pointed out that when children are fully stretched by cognitive demands they have little energy left for monitoring the procedure. It may be that some of our procedures are too demanding for the children and their monitoring skills cannot develop as a consequence. These points will be considered more fully in the discussion on therapeutic intervention. So far as identification is concerned we may summarise the cognitive aspect as follows:

1. Children who show delay in the acquisition of all aspects of language may be at risk for cognitive impairment.
2. Children who show evidence of cognitive impairment will be at risk for language delay and may be at risk for language disorders.
3. Delay in the emergence of symbolic play may herald either or both of the above conditions.

4. Language disorder may be heralded by a drop in the achievements of children previously showing average attainments on intelligence testing.
5. Language disorder may be indicated if children show considerable variability and quick fatigue in cognitive tasks.
6. Language disorder is more likely to be associated with inconsistency and variability in learning than is overall cognitive impairment and is also more likely to be modality specific.

Environmental risk factors

The identification of language disorders must involve examination of the factors in the child's environment that impede his learning of his native language. Attention must be paid to class and cultural considerations and the way in which these interact with biological risk factors. It has been stated many times that the factors that place children at risk for language disorder are compounds and not single entities. Children are placed at biological risk if they are born prematurely, if they are small for dates and if they are born to mothers who have taken drugs, smoked or drunk to excess during pregnancy. Poorly nourished, tired and worried mothers are far less likely to produce healthy infants than are those who are well cared for and well endowed. The materially developed countries of the western world have reason to be very concerned about the numbers of infants being born into financially deprived environments and also into environments that are polluted and unhealthy.

Children born at biological risk may be further affected in their development by parental attitudes. Poorly educated parents are less able to take advantage of what is offered in the way of health care than those who are well read and well informed. Mothers who are chronically tired and harassed will not have the time and energy to enjoy their babies and to interact with them in the positive way that will prepare them for communication through language. Many infants at biological risk are the products of teenage pregnancies. Very young mothers may have emotional needs of their own that are too strong to allow them to see their infants as individual beings with needs peculiar to themselves. Environmental risks to child development can best be viewed within a cumulative framework. We should start from first principles, that infants thrive best when they are healthy, well cared for, wanted and enjoyed. Skuse (1991) argues convincingly that it is not only cognitive but also physical growth that is affected by an under-stimulating, neglectful environment. The association between failure to thrive physically and failure to develop language at the normal rate has been demonstrated. Skuse emphasises the point that this relationship is most pronounced where there is a with-holding of the normal affection and warmth offered by a parent to his/her child in addition to a lack of stimulation.

Sensory deprivation

Severe sensory deprivation that occurs when children are reared in severely abnormal circumstances will surely prevent the acquisition of language. The case most frequently cited in the literature of language pathology, is that of Genie (Curtiss, 1977). Such tragic children cannot yield clear-cut evidence as to the effects of language deprivation alone because their chronic malnutrition prevents normal brain development.

Children learning more than one language

If ever there was evidence needed for the tremendous plasticity and capacity for reorganisation in the developing brain, then surely the young child's ability to learn more than one language simultaneously, with incredible facility compared with the lumbering adult learner, must provide it. Normally developing children with intact auditory and cognitive mechanisms can achieve bilingual status with consummate ease, switching from one language to another, and occasionally in the course of development, switching from one to another in one utterance (code-switching). Abudarham (1987) rejects the out-dated notion that learning two languages can have an adverse effect on speech and language development. Obviously if a child is exposed to a second language (L2) after he has commenced speaking in a first language, then he will lag behind his monoglot L2 peers, until such time as he has had the chance to catch up. The identification of the language-impaired child rests on his ability to communicate in his first language. The cooperation of speech and language therapists and co-workers (who have access to the numerous languages and dialects used in the UK's minorities) is essential here, in order to identify children who are at risk for learning any language.

Social class

The multicultural society is more topical in professional discussion among speech and language therapists than is social class. The latter was the focus of much interest during the 1960s when Bernstein's ideas were widely commented upon and widely misconstrued. It was then considered likely that children who were brought up in working-class environments were at a disadvantage compared with those middle-class children who had been exposed to a richer and more formal language experience during their formative years. This was partly because the child was likely to be educated by middle-class professionals no matter what his background. Children coming from middle-class backgrounds were therefore deemed to have considerable early advantages. The permanent effect of early language disadvantage or difference (see Edwards, JR, 1979) is now disproved in general terms. However, children who lack language stimulation in the sense of encouragement and enrichment are more likely to be delayed in language acquisition than are their linguistically privileged peers. This becomes a matter of some importance when instruments for language screening are being propagated.

Language opportunity and mother–child interaction

It is generally reported that children who lack opportunity to talk with adults or who have to compete continually for adult attention may show language delay. Evidence is yielded by both twin studies (Savic, 1980) and by the literature on social deprivation (Edwards, JR, 1979). One important variable in conducting research into language delay is the number of children in the home who are under 18 years of age. The British multicentre survey (Edwards, M, 1984) found that children with one or more siblings were over-represented in its sample when compared with the normal population distribution. Youngest children formed the majority of referrals. This finding was constant across all age groups within the sample range (3–6). The study did not find a higher incidence of referrals from one-parent families or from families where the mother was employed outside the home. It is not possible to draw firm conclusions from these findings in the absence of information about child-minding arrangements.

Another aspect of interest is that of mother–child matching in the development of language strategies. Bruner (1983a, b) describes some early work on infant language learning. The mother is noted as capitalising upon an object or activity that attracts the infant's attention. She establishes a joint referent for herself and her infant and makes this the focus of language, naming and describing. The development of this behaviour provides the language scaffolding through which the child can master linguistic forms by which to communicate experience. Bruner posits that the existence of a complex supportive language network, or Language Support System, makes possible the operation of genetically determined language devices.

A considerable literature has developed about the mother's behaviour in facilitating the language development of her child. A number of studies (Snow, 1972; Bloom, 1973; Snow and Ferguson, 1977) have shown how mothers adjust their speech to the developing abilities of their language-learning infants. Mothers produce speech that is syntactically simple, redundant and semantically related to topics of interest to young children. This simplified register has come to be known as `motherese'. Authors have challenged the idea that children do in fact learn best from simplified data (Gleitman, Newport and Gleitman, 1984) and it has been suggested that language is most helpfully learned from data that mirror the range and complexities of the language system. Others (Furrow and Nelson, 1986) affirm the opposite view. The argument is

obviously of more than academic interest to speech and language therapists both as regards the causal and the remedial aspects of language
delay. It has been demonstrated (Lieven, 1978) that there are conspicuous differences in the response parents make to conversationally adept
and conversationally inept children. Handicapped children who cannot
signal their intentions nor generate statements cannot stimulate adults
to respond. Thus communication breaks down and with it the possibility
of language growth. However, this is a long way from saying that normal
children may become language deficient because their mothers fail to
talk to them in an appropriate way. Many suppositions about factors
making for language delay have been made without knowledge of individual variation. The question of language style and of style matching
has yet to find a place in the literature of language therapy. Clinicians do
not, as a matter of routine, analyse the language of adults when interacting with the infants and children in their care. We may hope to see
more emphasis upon the dyad in future investigation. Conti-Ramsden
(1987, 1993) has drawn attention to the importance of placing any
dyadic analyses within the context in which they occur if a true picture is
to emerge. Such analyses could then lead to interactive language therapy
making use of each partner's contribution.

We will now turn from those factors that are important in identification to the manner in which the identification takes place.

Prediction of language abilities: transient or persistent?

One of the most difficult tasks for the speech and language clinician
working with young children is to predict which children will go on to
have *confirmed language impairments* and which children have *transient language delays*. As yet there is still no proven accurate means of
making such conclusive decisions. If it were possible to identify those
children with long-term needs accurately it would serve several
purposes: one would be confident in reassuring parents of the prognosis; the needs of children could be immediately met; and, in principle,
the provision of services might be more accurately targeted at those children whose need is greatest. At present, early identification of children
with language delay in speech and language clinics is followed by a
period of advice and review. Does the literature provide any research
evidence which will guide the decision-making process regarding the
outcome for these children?

Firstly, the evidence from familial studies suggests that the truly
language-impaired child is very likely to have affected relatives, which
makes this an imperative question in the case history. But this is not a
very reliable prognostic sign, because some very impaired children have
no family history. There do appear to be some implications for later
childhood, however. Tallal, Townsend, Curtiss and Wulfeck (1991)

showed that (Specific language impairment) children with a positive family history were less likely to do well on standardised tests of academic achievement than those without a positive family history.

Does the nature of the language delay help us to identify the child with persistent impairment from the one with transient impairment? Whitehurst and Fischel (1994) think that it does. In an influential paper they argue, from longitudinal data collected from children with developmental language delays, that the majority of these children will be within normal limits on language tests by the time they are 5 years old. Moreover, they put forward the view that *the child with an expressive delay only would be more likely to recover than the child with combined receptive-expressive problems*.

The work of Thal and her colleagues (Thal and Bates, 1988, Thal, Tobias and Morrison, 1991) goes some way to confirming the conclusions of Whitehurst and Fischel (1994). Thal, Tobias and Morrison (1991) followed up the group of late talkers identified by Thal and Bates in 1988. They discovered that some of the original subjects had caught up with respect to their language skills, but that a proportion remained 'truly delayed'. This sub-group turned out to have been poorer than the recovered group on early measures of gestural ability (which might be seen as a symbolic skill), and had been significantly delayed in verbal comprehension. Both Thal's work and that of Ellis Weismer, Murray-Branch and Miller (1994) suggest that *early (mean length of utterance) measures do not help to predict continued language delay*.

One cannot doubt the results that Whitehurst and his colleagues have found. However, these conclusions remain slightly dangerous for two reasons. One is that we know, as clinicians, that consideration of individual cases always takes priority, and that it may be unwise to adopt a policy of prioritisation from such group studies as this. Group studies obscure individual results. This is not a phenomenon restricted to language pathology. Related fields such as dyslexia have suffered from these difficulties of prediction for many years. There is also a paradox here. The most commonly identified form of persistent specific language impairment is the phonologic–syntactic disorder, or expressive language disorder (see Chapter 5). What do these children look like in their preschool years? Do they not present with just the very expressive language delays that Whitehurst and Fischel are keen to dismiss as transient? It would be expedient to be very cautious about their claims.

Of course Whitehurst and Fischel (1994) had found the same facts as had Bishop and Edmundson (1987a). That is that most children identified as language-delayed very early in life do recover to normal. However, 'some children with specific language delay go on to have learning or language impairments in the school years' (Whitehurst and Fischel, 1994), and it is these children whose needs are barely met by current service provision. Bishop and Edmundson looked at *all* the preschool children referred to speech and language therapists over a period of time. Had all of these children required long-term intervention the speech and language therapy services would have had to increase exponentially.

Are there factors in the preschool child that reliably predict whether there will be persistent impairment or not? Bishop and Edmundson (1987a) found that one of the best predictors of later language skill was a story retelling task (*The Bus Story*, Renfrew 1972). They also found that isolated impairments (say in phonology) had the best outcome, and that associated poor non-verbal skills generally indicated a poor outcome. Stark and Tallal (in McCauley, 1988) analysed data from 36 children with specific language impairment and discovered impressive associations between language measures and scores on perceptual motor tasks, including speech perception and fine motor skills. Sommers (1991) set out with the aim of predicting language abilities of children with developmental delays (i.e. not necessarily language specific) and found that language development was closely related to mental age and motor skills, in addition to other factors.

To summarise, the current state of research suggests that the worst-case scenario, in terms of prognosis for language, would be the child with:

1. borderline/low IQ;
2. poor story retelling skills;
3. poor comprehension/symbolic skills; and
4. family history of speech/language problems.

A better outcome would be predicted for:

1. normal/above average IQ;
2. circumscribed linguistic problem, usually phonology;
3. normal comprehension/symbolic skills; and
4. no family history.

Many clinicians will, from their working experience be able to think of individual children who flout these guidelines, and there is currently no case for accepting them as correct until more, well-controlled research has taken place.

Screening

Procedures for language screening must satisfy the ethical requirements laid down by the WHO (1980) and respected by all in health care as part of a health surveillance strategy. One absolute prerequisite is that the condition under identification is one that can be cured or mitigated; and the second is that procedures exist for cure or remediation. When children are screened for language disorders we must ensure that special education and therapy are available. The step between screening and remediation is diagnosis to determine whether a condition that is handicapping does indeed exist. Assessment is the fellow of diagnosis because this shows the extent of the handicapping features together with the strengths and abilities that accompany them.

To screen is to administer a simple procedure that will accurately pick out children who may need special services. A screen will separate out those children who need further investigation from those whose development and attainments are normal or who are not at risk for the condition under investigation. Screening procedures must be:

1. Economical both in time and materials.
2. Simple and capable of being replicated by other professional workers.
3. Comprehensive in the area of interest.
4. Sufficiently accurate to ensure a minimum of false positives and false negatives, that is to say that they should be capable of detecting children who have the condition and not identifying those who do not.
5. Cost effective–the condition to be detected must affect a large number of children whose progress as a result of early detection will save special medical and educational expenses such as to balance the costs of screening.

Any kind of identification procedure creates anxiety. People exposing themselves to medical screening of any kind must understand the consequences of identification. It is highly important therefore that they should have immediate access to investigative and counselling services. However, they also have a responsibility to prepare themselves for screening by finding out as much as they can beforehand and making sure that they are able to tolerate an adverse result. If the condition is serious enough to demand early identification and investigation, it is sufficient to cause disquiet. If it can cause disquiet, people must be prepared for it. Because screening preschool children raises many issues that are not present in school-age screening, the two populations will be dealt with separately.

Preschool screening: infants and young children

Language milestones have always been incorporated into developmental screening or developmental surveillance because they contain so much information as to the infant's sensory, motor and cognitive abilities. We have seen a change of emphasis in that physicians are being asked to screen for language impairment not only as an indicator of other handicaps (deafness, severe learning impairment) but as a handicapping condition in its own right. The recognition of this claim has caused some paediatricians in the USA to develop their own screening instruments for language (Capute et al., 1986). These seek to extend the developmental screening test most frequently used, the Denver Developmental Scale (Frankenburg et al., 1981), which lacks sufficient early points on language development. In the UK, the hearing screening of all infants by health visitors contributes one essential element to the identification of potential language impairment, (but the regular application of developmental screening is now erratic as a result of national policy changes (Law and Pollard, 1994)).

The development of language in infancy and early childhood is now well charted and the factors that contribute to it are also known. Behaviours that indicate that the language acquisition process is taking place can therefore be recorded and used as screening points. During the second and third year of life, screening can employ one procedure, e.g. naming, to demonstrate evidence of both speech and hearing ability. The age at which a particular behaviour emerges is left purposely unspecified within a couple of months because too arbitrary a determination is out of keeping with infant variability and can cause anxiety. Comparison of infant developmental scales devised by different authors shows a number of differences within a couple of months on both receptive and expressive language items (Byers Brown, Bendersky and Chapman, 1986; Byers Brown, 1987).

The difficulty in screening infants for possible language delay is to find items that have good predictive validity. Infant development shows both continuities and discontinuities. One skill may precede another but does not necessarily predict another. To say that a child will be delayed in speech because he showed little use of expressive jargon at 11 months is highly unwise. On the other hand an infant who shows no repetitive babble at all during the first year is outside the limit of normal variation.

The developmental outlines tabled give a broad view of progress in receptive and expressive skills but do not give any information upon interaction, a vital component of language development.

The only exception is the item 'reciprocal vocalisation' at 2–3 months. However, most early developmental and language scales add some items to gauge the extent of a child's general responsiveness and his ability to respond to and to initiate play (peek-a-boo, pat-a-cake). It can be seen that the kind of stimulation in the home would play a decisive part in the child's behaviour in this area.

The object in propagating screening instruments is to allow for the detection of possible abnormality without requiring individual judgement from the person administering the instrument. To invite the administrator to look for mitigating factors or to use his own discretion in the acceptance of a response is to invite disaster. People who carry out screening programmes are not necessarily, experts in all aspects of child development. In the UK, the health visitor is an

Table 2.2 Hearing acuity – comprehension: Development of communication skills 1

0 (months) 1	2	3	4	5	6	7	8	9	10	11	12
Responds to sounds by startle	Eye blink Eye widening Arousal from sleep Reduction of activity	Responds differently to angry/ friendly, familiar/ unfamiliar voices	Rudimentary head turn to side of sound		Head turn to noise Turns to own name	Localises to side and indirectly below		Appears to recognise names of self and family	Responds to 'no'	Localises to side and directly below	Responds to request plus gesture
						Turns or smiles to 'Where's Daddy' etc.					

Table 2.3 Speech motor–linguistic activity: Development of communication skills 2

0 (months) 1	2	3	4	5	6	7	8	9	10	11	12
Reflexive crying Vegetative sounds	Reciprocal vocalisation Cooing Laughter Vocal play Raspberry			Repetitive babbling	-------Variegated babbling-------			-------Expressive jargon-------		Intentional vocalising	Sounds and words
	Vowel-type sounds Differentiated crying										

Table 2.4 Receptive and expressive language: Development of communication

12 (months)	14	16	18	20	22	24	26	28	30	32	34	36
Recognises familiar rounds	*Looks at objects named*			*Recognises body parts*		*Listens to meaning* *Points to objects named*		*Obtaining information primarily through language*				
uses names and function words, e.g. there		Dramatic growth in spoken vocabulary		Two word utterances		Uses different linguistic elements to vary meaning			Sentences expanding in length and complexity			
		Words with intonation and jargon				Word endings						
		Initiates communication				Prepositions						
						Word combinations						

invaluable investigator and one who can carry out a number of procedures that are helpful in the identification of language delay. But the
criteria for failure and referral must be clear and unambiguous. Such
criteria are easier to establish with regard to hearing and comprehension than they are with regard to speech. Perhaps, if there has to be a
partiality, it is much safer to have it this way because hearing and
comprehension are so vital for the child's social, cognitive, emotional
and educational development. Any item on the first year developmental chart for hearing and comprehension (Table 2.2) which the
child fails should warrant follow-up. Key screening items can therefore
be selected with regard to an unequivocal nature of the behaviour and
the ease with which it can be evoked.

Parent report

Screening studies have also sought information on the relative predictive power of parents when compared with workers administering a
screening instrument. Parents might be asked whether or not they
were concerned about their children's speech or hearing, and the
results compared with the sensitivity of the screening instrument in
terms of true and false positives. Although it may be suggested that
questioning parents would be as valuable as early childhood
screening, it does not suggest that parents necessarily volunteer the
information. To respond 'Yes' when asked if you are concerned is a
different matter from taking your child to the doctor or speech clinic
because of this concern. As Law, (1992) points out, parents may have
very different expectations of their children than professionals do, and
this would be especially significant if the children who were most at
risk are the children whose parents have the lowest expectations.
Much of the value of a screening instrument lies in the prompt it gives
to primary health workers to direct attention towards significant areas
of development. If all children were seen regularly for developmental
surveillance during early childhood, and if the relationship between
physician and parent were such that easy discussion was a feature of
the interview, formal screening would not be necessary. The onus
would be upon professionals concerned with speech, language and
hearing development to make sure that up-to-date knowledge on
important areas was fed through to those responsible for primary
health care. Unfortunately, children who fall through surveillance nets
are very likely to be disadvantaged children who may be the most at
risk. The 'inverse care' law operates here, according to Hall (1992), i.e.
those who need the most help are the least likely to apply for it.
  Speech and language therapists in the UK have cooperated with
paediatricians in reviewing developmental screening policy on a regular
basis (Levitt and Muir, 1983; Lindsay, 1984). The following points are

those which may offer the safest guidelines at this stage of our knowledge. Failure indicates the need for follow-up:

6–12 months   Infant responds to sound. Mother expresses no concern about
                     hearing. Infant coos, laughs, reciprocates vocally.

12 months   Infant vocalises to sound. Mother expresses no concern about
                     hearing. Infant vocalises and babbles.

12–18 months   Infant locates sound source; carries out one-step commands.
                     Mother expresses no concern about hearing. Infant uses some
                     words spontaneously and correctly.

18–24 months   Infant follows simple instruction without gesture; points to at least
                     one body part when named. Mother expresses no concern about
                     hearing. Infant verbally expresses wants; steadily increases
                     number of words used; uses two-word combination around 24
                     months. Mother expresses no concern about speech.

This constitutes a simple yet fairly comprehensive screen. Any other
signs that place the child at risk (prematurity, genetic hearing loss) should
ensure that the child receives a more thorough professional examination
at 3-monthly or 6-monthly intervals. The relationship of these early identification procedures to prophylaxis will be discussed in the next chapter.

Some screening procedures have focused upon productive vocabulary and the ability to combine words between 24 and 30 months. It has
been demonstrated that parents find it easier to recognise the words
their children say when shown a vocabulary checklist than when asked
to recall them spontaneously during an interview. The procedure advocated by Rescorla (1989, 1993) has much to recommend it. The parent is
asked to indicate, on a comprehensive vocabulary checklist, all the
words the child uses spontaneously and then asked to write down examples of sentences, phrases or word combinations. The child fails if he has
less than 50 words and no two-word combinations. Dixon, Kot and Law
(1988) describe a preliminary version of a screening procedure developed with an inner-city population for use with children of 2.5 years.
The content of the test was based around that of the Derbyshire
Language Scheme, and incorporated items to screen comprehension
and expression, using simple toys and some pictures. The evaluation of
a procedure such as this is essential, but time-consuming, as one has to
identify redundant items and decide whether the test really does identify
the children who are truly language-delayed. Experience of designing
and implementing such procedures indicates *the speech and language
therapist has a critical role to play in the child surveillance process.*

The practice of screening for very early language impairment has
undergone radical reorganisation in the UK. The Health for All Children

report (Hall, 1991) created a rationale, whether by accident or design, for health services to cut back on the costly business of screening for speech and language delay (the forerunner of developmental language disorders), to the extent that some regions now have little screening carried out at all. Given the significance of early language delay in the detection of a range of developmental deficits with long-term implications for intervention and special education being a well established fact, this is a difficult develop-ment to comprehend. The rationale may have arisen from Hall's reflec-tions on the fact that because there is 'no absolute definition of SLI' there can be .... 'no watertight screening test' (Hall, 1992, p. 247). The consensus appears to be that, whereas this has some truth in it, *the overall outcome has been most unhelpful*. Law and Pollard (1994) argue very strongly for the continuation of early screening, on the premise that intervention in the early years is a most effective way of preventing later education and social difficulties. The withdrawal of a programme of surveillance, with no evident means of a replacement scheme, or even a pragmatic strategy for picking these children up through parent education, has *profound impli-cations* for the identification of early language delay and language disorder (in addition to related developmental conditions), and has gone largely unheralded by the speech and language therapy profession.

Screening for the school population

As the child approaches school age, screening for language delay or disorders becomes easier in that there are many more markers. Normal 4-year-olds converse and narrate by means of intelligible speech. Phonology and grammar have been sufficiently well documented through child language research to generate reliable screening guide-lines. It will be for the speech and language therapy and education services to decide what kind of identification system to put into effect. No quick screen will pick up the subtle problems of comprehension or interaction that indicate language disorders of the semantic–pragmatic type. The quicker the test, the more it tends to focus upon articulation as a criterion. Those responsible may therefore decide that rather than institute a one-off screening procedure, they will invest in teacher-based identification procedures. The ethical considerations still apply. Once a child has been identified as being at risk he must be given diagnostic and remedial services. If these are not available educational authorities will not wish to have possible problems identified. On the other hand without some kind of screening of the school population, the need for services cannot be calculated and the services planned.

The Association for All Speech Impaired Children has produced a screening test for language impairment, specifically designed for admin-istration by teachers (AFASIC, 1991). It therefore has a dual purpose: the identification of language-impaired children and the education of teachers in this complex subject. The instructions state that the child should be reasonably well known to the teacher before the test is administered. A period of observation prior to administration may be necessary. The reason for these injunctions becomes clear when the test is studied. Information is sought on all major areas pertaining to language disorder, motor, cognitive and play behaviour as well as language measures. A profile is compiled that will then indicate the main areas of deficit and strength. The test takes time to prepare for and to administer and yet in no way precludes the need for full assessment once the child is identified as at risk. Teachers who lack recourse to specialists in language disorders may find such a profile gives them enough help in working with the child to justify the time spent. Others, who have more ready access to other services, may prefer to follow a simple list of questions such as that compiled by Beveridge and Conti-Ramsden (1987). Samples are: 'Does the pupil often misunderstand simple instructions? .... not seem fully to understand logical correctives? .... avoid tasks and situations involving language?' The teacher may then request further investigation or not according to the pattern of response.

Identification of later language learning difficulties

Language growth represents a slow, gradual continuum of change and modification. During the process there are periods of acceleration and periods where nothing much seems to be happening. These periods may represent reorganisations that will then be followed by further growth. Children will be presented with educational challenges and increased cognitive demands during their school careers. It is likely that some of these demands cannot be met by children whose earlier language abilities appeared adequate. Reasons are indicated in the earlier discussion on maturational lag. Teachers need to be sensitive to the effects of new language demands upon children who were at any time delayed in speech because their time-scale of growth may be different from their peers. They may have longer plateau periods and less acceleration between plateaux. Children who have shown early, slight, motor difficulties in combination with delayed language may break down again at a much later age when demands for writing at speed are made.

Other manifestations of language inadequacy might be unruly and disruptive behaviour in class and lack of participation in group discussions. Children who find that they cannot follow group instructions are likely to react in this way. Children who become aware of differences between their own ability to absorb and generate information through language and those of their peers may become obstreperous or withdrawn. Truanting offers a way out for some and illness for others. There are, of course, other reasons why older children and adolescents start to rebel against their teachers or against the school system in general. Nevertheless, language disability must always be considered when such behaviour follows an early history of speech delay.

The most helpful way in which speech and language therapists can contribute to the identification of these later difficulties is to ensure that all early problems of spoken language are well documented. Snowling (1985b) observes that speech and language therapists, working at the interface of medicine and education, in preschool and primary school play a crucial role in the prevention, early detection, assessment and management of children's written language difficulties. She believes that speech and language therapists should be involved at every stage in identifying, monitoring and, where appropriate, treating the specific educational needs of individuals who, if not in their care, have at some stage passed through it. Stackhouse (1985), writes about the relationship between phonetic speech difficulties and subsequent spelling problems. Ideally, speech and language therapists should keep under review children with poor phoneme–grapheme conversion skills because, although their speech may have improved, they are at risk for spelling problems. The extent to which this can be done will, of course, depend upon the numbers of children involved and the extent of speech and language therapy provision.

It can be seen that the identification of language disorder, whether latent or present, is a *multidisciplinary function*. Although the alarm may be given by one person, parent or professional, that alarm will be given much more readily and accurately if a lot of what is known by specialists can be filtered through to those who are in daily contact with the child. Specialist knowledge will itself be increased and buttressed by the feedback received from those whose interest they have succeeded in alerting. Specialists also have a responsibility to see that the child's difficulties and abilities are well documented and that this documentation is available to those who inherit the child as a pupil. The fact that children may receive speech and language therapy under the auspices of the health service can prevent those in education becoming aware of the child's history. Breakdown can also occur if a child moves into another school district or simply moves from primary to secondary school. Such breakdown can only be prevented by vigilance on the part of everyone involved.

Chapter 3
Prevention

Summary

This chapter looks again at the factors that may place a child at risk for language disorder, in order to see how their impact can be minimised. It considers the general nature of prevention through public and professional education. Specific reference is made to a number of prophylactic measures that may be advocated. Suggestions for parent guidance are given. Particular attention is paid to the ways in which secondary features of the disorder can be prevented. Examples both of useful books and good practice are given. Speech and language precursors are discussed in some detail in relation both to detection and prevention of abnormality.

The more we know about how language disorders develop the greater becomes our responsibility to try to prevent them. Professional growth may be judged by the way it moves from correction to overall management. But before we consider what overall management might entail, we need to deliberate on what is meant by prevention. Can language disorders be prevented from developing? If as we have argued some language impairments are organically constituted, then surely prevention is an unattainable goal for some children. We must simply wait for the disorder to unfold. Or are there some children whose predisposition to language impairment might be overcome by removal of the adverse additional factors that conspire to push the child into overt language disorder. Can language delay be prevented from becoming language disorder? Can we adopt what Law (1992) terms 'an approach of damage limitation', i.e. the development of further symptoms, by working through families and the environment, rather than on the child. Can existing language impairments be managed in such a way as to preclude the evolution of more deviant profiles?

The principles of prevention

There are few speech pathologists who have taken an interest in the general principles of prevention, Michael Marge of the USA being one of

54

the best know (Marge, 1984). Marge distinguishes between primary, secondary and tertiary prevention, which we will redefine here.

Primary prevention

This is the elimination or inhibition of the onset or development by altering susceptibility or reducing exposure for susceptible persons. An example would be the protection from ear infections that might lead to hearing loss and delayed language development.

Secondary prevention

This is early detection which may lead to elimination of the disorder, retardation of its progress and prevention of further complications. Early hearing screening is an instance of this. If a conductive hearing loss were found, the infant could receive medical or surgical treatment to reverse the disease process, and language stimulation to promote language learning.

Tertiary prevention

This constitutes the reduction of a disability through the promotion of effective function. Should the infant's hearing loss prove to be irreversible, means to aid residual hearing and to teach language must be put into effect. If successful they should allow the child to benefit from education to the full and to develop socially and emotionally to his full potential.

Speech and language therapists must be concerned with prophylaxis, which can be seen as the taking of an active step towards prevention. They may not be able to shield a child from ear infections but they can see that he is protected from adverse linguistic consequences through efficient hearing testing and language guidance. Some of the means they can employ have already been indicated. For example, one of the major practices of secondary prevention is the mass screening of persons without symptoms.

Language delays and disorders are themselves secondary to biological and environmental conditions. So in considering how we can prevent these delays and disorders, we are faced with a number of factors outside our control. Here we can only hope to intervene effectively at the secondary or tertiary level. There are other conditions where we may hope to prevent the language abnormality from occurring in the first place. The points upon which we can impact to alter factors adverse to language development will be discussed together with the practicalities of prophylaxis. Tertiary prevention will be considered more fully in Chapter 7 because it is part of language intervention.

Public and professional awareness

The first part of any campaign for primary or secondary prevention is the raising of the general consciousness about deleterious practice and how to avoid it. Infants are at biological risk for language disorders as for other developmental problems if they are conceived by sick parents, damaged in utero, malnourished, small for dates and preterm. They are at risk if they are born into less than optimal environments and under-nourished. All educated people who are able to inform themselves on these points have a duty to campaign on the side of a healthy society. Speech and language therapists are one of the professional groups that see the consequences to children of any kind of abuse; they will there-fore wish to associate themselves with all movements designed to improve infant health and to protect children from the consequences of adult ignorance and short-sightedness. Their direct responsibilities are for communication and language.

One of the authors of this text (BBB) took part in an exercise in New Jersey (USA) designed to promote an efficient, coordinated scheme through which to identify infants and young children who were at risk for, or suffering from, communication disorders. Preliminary investiga-tion suggested that there were a number of systems of services in which such children could be involved. These service systems comprised hospital or diagnostic centre, community clinic, and maternal and child health programmes. The children could also be identified through one of several parallel child-care systems including state efforts to implement the Education for all Handicapped Children Act, State Developmental Disabilities Programs, Head Start and Early Intervention Services either at home or centre based. There were also a number of facilities devel-oped by voluntary health agencies and private practitioners in paedi-atrics, audiology, psychology and speech-language pathology. There seemed little point in attempting to add to these facilities. The research team therefore determined to promote, augment and seek to coordinate those service systems that were already in use. Through careful study of the way in which the systems were being used, we hoped to find out what lay behind the general complaint that children were not being referred early enough to benefit fully from speech, language and hearing services.

Underlying the research team's efforts was the rationale that because no one single profession is responsible for all aspects of care, successful management must involve the coordination of different aspects of professional responsibility. Thus, once more we were drawn to look at the systems within which professionals worked. Attention was also directed towards parent and public education because this creates the climate within which systems of care may flourish. The aims of the project were as follows:

- To improve the general level of public and professional awareness.
- To improve the skills of those involved in primary identification.
- To offer more resources to those concerned with diagnosis and management.
- To identify specific weaknesses in the identification and referral systems.

All these points are directly concerned with prevention: primary, secondary and tertiary.

The project

The target population was children aged 0–4 in a four-county area of New Jersey. The research team first announced its intention to promote better identification of children at risk for communication disorders through newspaper and state professional bulletins, radio and television programmes. It invited cooperation and appealed for information on existing facilities. Special meetings were held with the New Jersey Speech and Hearing Association and with other organisations serving handicapped children. There was also full discussion with the New Jersey State Department of Health followed by cooperative investigation carried out jointly by the research team and by those in charge of the Newborn Hearing Program for High Risk Infants. As a result, two major studies were mounted by the research team, which was based in the Department of Paediatrics of the State Medical School. The first study examined the Newborn Screening Program which had reported a compliance rate of only 17%. It was considered that if children known to be at risk attracted such a poor screening response, there would be little point in attempting to develop further programmes until the reasons were known.

Table 3.1 shows the deficiencies revealed and the remedies proposed. The deficiencies arose mainly from lack of communication between the various groups (i.e. administrative, professional and

Table 3.1 Investigation of Newborn Hearing Program for High Risk Infants (Study 1)

Deficiencies revealed	Remedies initiated
Parents inadequately informed regarding:	Parent education
1. Reasons for child's registration	Public and professional information campaign
2. Procedures	Revised criteria for inclusion
3. Financial assistance	Additional subsidised assessment centres
Physicians not convinced regarding:	Screening training
1. Value of programme	Entire programme revised by State
2. Reasons for inclusion	Department of Health
3. Results of own screening	
4. Effectiveness of early diagnosis	

parental) that were involved. However, there was a general lack of faith in the screening process that needed to be tackled directly. The remedies proved to be effective as was indicated by a considerable increase in the compliance rate at the end of the next year. Regular revision of the programme should ensure that this continues and improves still further.

The second study was undertaken to establish the identity of those professionals who assessed young children for communication disorders. Professionals in the USA command a very wide range of employers when compared with the UK where the National Health service (NHS) is the major employer, at least of speech and language therapists. Private practice was particularly prosperous in New Jersey. Table 3.2 shows the deficiencies revealed and remedies initiated. A conspicuous finding was the dearth of assessment instruments available for very young children as distinct from those of between 2;6 and 4 years of age. From this study we were able to calculate the number of children in different age groups who reached the assessors. We learned more about referral routes and the conditions most likely to prompt referrals. As a consequence we were able to decide where to concentrate our attack in the attempt to improve identification. The establishment of a baseline number of referrals for the different ages meant that we were also able to measure our own efforts by the subsequent increase in numbers. These efforts included a number of training sessions for paediatricians and nurses together with presentations at professional conferences and a variety of medical and educational centres.

Table 3.2 Identification of assessors in early child communication (Study 2)

Deficiencies revealed	Remedies initiated
1. Delay in referral	Continuing education for primary care
2. Delay in assessment after referral	personnel and for those who assess
3. Inadequate assessment instruments	Promotion of new techniques
4. Inappropriate assessment instruments	Propagation of research findings on
5. Lack of parental interest	development of communication skills
6. Lack of services for 0–2-year-olds	Parent education
	New sites for screening and assessment
	Revision of assessment tools
	Research into communicative behaviour of 0–2-year-olds

The research team carried out its own studies into early communication development and as a result suggested a number of items that were then incorporated into both screening and assessment procedures. Language items were added to the hearing items that constituted the main follow-up procedure in communication screening for infants at risk due to prematurity or genetic factors. The overall result was to reduce the waiting time between first identification and subsequent assessment for all children, but particularly for the younger ones, and

Table 3.3 Conditions and circumstances leading to deterioration of screening programmes

Conditions	Causes	Remedies initiated
Time pressure	Over scheduling Emergencies Number and variety of tasks to be accomplished Financial profit	Task analysis Elimination of redundant and unnecessary procedures Assistance from research personnel in conducting screening
Lack of knowledge	Training in procedures only without teaching of principles and background Complex nature of communicative development	Regular demonstration and discussion of cases In-service training Distribution of reading material Research team available for reference
Staff change	Unsatisfactory conditions Inadequate remuneration Natural wastage	Beyond the efforts of research staff except as above to improve morale
Lack of feedback	Parents fail to follow through Screening personnel not informed of results of assessment	Continuous and sustained effort to improve flow of information Parent interviews Professional conferences Preparation of suitable forms of exchange of information
Low morale	Associated with all the factors recorded above	All measures indicated above plus expression of appreciation

Some of the remedies put into effect by research staff could not be maintained beyond the life of the project. Others were incorporated into the system and continue to be effective. A main contribution of the research was to indicate the extent to which a system is vulnerable to breakdown and to recommend review procedures.

considerably to increase the number of appropriate referrals. Once more, it is considered that the procedures should continue to promote better practice.

It became apparent during the studies described above, that screening programmes will deteriorate unless very serious efforts are made to maintain them. Table 3.3 indicates some of the factors leading to deterioration in some of the New Jersey programmes. They have their counterparts elsewhere. Indeed, the point of describing the New Jersey project is to draw attention to the counterparts that exist in other countries. Systems of health care may differ but the needs and behaviour of people working in them will be the same. The success of the research project was, of course, very much due to the funds it had available to produce materials and to help mount activities. Nevertheless, the most important factor was almost certainly staff enthusiasm and time spent with the primary care personnel. When a research staff member was present, identification of communication problems became a focus of interest. Once she left, time became swallowed up by other things. The moral is very clear. We cannot mount programmes to identify and to prevent conditions occurring unless there are funds to maintain them and unless there are people who have a major interest and continuing investment in them. Another point to be made is that speech and language therapists must find ways of having an impact upon the systems controlling health care and education if prophylactic measures are to be developed.

Prevention by detection

If early detection of language delay is to be a serious venture, allies must be sought among those professionals involved in developmental surveillance: the family doctor, the paediatrician, the health visitor and community nurse. In the UK, the health visitor has long been trained in hearing screening, among other activities. He or she is consequently in a very good position to carry out any other procedures related to communication development. Ward (1984) describes a study in which health visitors were chosen to administer questionnaires about auditory behaviour because parents were familiar with the health visitors' interest in hearing and would not become anxious when questioned by them.

The success of health visitors in making appropriate referrals to the speech and language therapist has already been indicated in this text. An essential part of any in-service programme through which to train health visitors and other workers would be the demonstration of early delays and deviations and possible outcomes. When referrals are made, full information on the results of the assessment should be fed back as speedily as possible. When this is not done, enthusiasm wanes and potential skills are wasted. Because health visitors are likely to be in demand for a number of important duties, it is obviously essential not to add to their activities without giving them the job satisfaction to which they are entitled.

Screening and first identification procedures should be brief and easy to administer as has been emphasised in Chapter 2. Nevertheless, there are minimum standards that must be met. An attempt was made in New Jersey to enlist the aid of community nurses in Well Baby clinics and this immediately threw up the difficulty inherent in almost every baby clinic site. Some of the places in which the nurses worked were extremely noisy and crowded, and there was almost invariably pressure of time. In addition to their own busy schedules, the nurses had to consider mothers with a number of fretful small children, all anxious to get home. There was scarcely ever a refusal to cooperate, only an understandable temptation to put on one side any matters that were not causing anxiety. Professionals are continually forced to compromise between their own interests and those of the parents, but there are many instances where compromise is not possible. It is far better that the procedures should not be attempted at all and this fact recorded in the case history than that the procedure should be carried out too cursorily with the risk of an inaccurate result.

The preventive aspect of early identification is its strongest weapon and this should always be fully explained. One screening programme that was carried out among a largely middle-class professional White population was ill received because the parents perceived it as an assessment procedure and considered that it did not do justice to their children's abilities. If screening is to be used continually as a preventive measure, we cannot afford to have the procedures fall into disrepute. As a means of educating public opinion, it may not be the best way to proceed. If the intention is to locate children who are at risk for a condition known to be prevalent and punitive, general screening may well be advocated. The important thing is to use this vehicle, as all others, with judgement and in a spirit of enthusiastic realism.

As the child enters into a larger world, he or she has more opportunity both to practise language skills and to reveal language deficiencies. Instead of the mother and health care professionals being the only judges of the child's attainment, there are likely to be nursery teachers, nursery aids, play group managers, day care centre staff and others who have the opportunity to look at an individual child in the company of his or her peers. Helping a non-verbal child to experience and enjoy language and to try to communicate are very reasonable goals within small social groups. Where the number of children is large and the number of adults small, no great benefits can be expected. However, even in these cases identification of communication delays is possible, particularly when there is good working contact with the speech and language therapy service. Where identification is possible, some prophylactic measures may be applied.

A child's differing environment may have a role to play in altering susceptibility. For example, if a child is born into a family where there is a tendency towards delayed language, the child's parents may request his or her early admission to a nursery that offers more stimulating play and musical materials than the home can provide. The child may also receive more communicative challenge. Conversely, nursery staff may observe that a child becomes more confused and tired than his peers when verbally stimulated. They may suggest that the child spends more time with a single care-giver who can give him more individual guidance until his attention and listening skills improve.

A young child joining a nursery or play group for the first time becomes prone to infections. If a child has already experienced a number of episodes of otitis media in infancy he is at increased risk for further episodes in childhood. Nursery staff may be very helpful in noting a child's response to sounds and advising parents of the need to seek medical opinion.

Children who lack communicative opportunity or communicative effort may benefit considerably from an extension of their environment. If they have to communicate in order to satisfy needs or gratify wishes, they will try to do so. Observant adults may note whether the attempts to communicate increase the child's skills or cause distress. They can give help, or withhold it, in the light of their judgement. Thus a new situation is one that provides opportunity to detect, support, report and possibly teach necessary skills.

Prevention by information

To give people useful information is not necessarily to make them act more wisely but it does give them the opportunity. Because so much of what we know about good language development technique has come from our observation of parents, it is only right that we feed back to parents the results of our observations. Outstandingly, we have learned that no one theory of language development based upon formal linguistic studies or single cognitive or perceptual systems can suffice to explain language development (Trevarthen, Murray and Hubley, 1981): `Infants communicate by using all their faculties in sensitive dependence on both the human and the practical, usable environment'. The infant, although seemingly highly dependent upon his mother for language nourishment, has been shown to be capable of exerting considerable control, even in very early exchanges. His gradual mastery of language is part of a dynamic, interactive process in which his behaviour stimulates the mother towards skilful support and education (see Lewis and Freedle, 1973; Lewis, 1977; Trevarthen, Murray and Hubley, 1981; Trevarthen and Marwick, 1986).

Trevarthen and Marwick (1986) point out that the intrinsic motivation of the expressive and receptive processes in the child's mind is so strong that it is unlikely that his behaviour will simply reflect the frequency of occurrence of particular items in the mother's activity. Parents then should be reassured that they are not responsible for teaching the child to talk by following any particular method. Nor are they responsible for any slowness he may show in talking simply because they have failed to indulge in any one speech-oriented activity during the early months of life. They will only be responsible if they fail to supply a happy relationship for the baby with a person easily and frequently available to him.

Some of the effects of our early discoveries on the importance of early language development may have been to over-emphasise the role of `mother-talk' simply as talk. Although mothers who are naturally chatty and expressive may greatly enjoy talking to their very young babies, others may not find it so easy. So the less exuberant mothers will read with relief that the quality of their responses, the way in which they react by smiling, touching and directing the infant's attention to objects of interest will serve the infant just as well. He does need to learn that he can have an effect upon his environment, that communicative effort brings rewards and that sustained response to visual and auditory experiences is enjoyable. The first two of these can only be learned with adult help. The third he will learn if adults refrain from interfering with his enjoyment by offering competing stimuli. At a somewhat later stage they will help by providing materials calculated to hold his interest and showing him how to attend to them.

Giving information about mother–child talk

As babies grow into toddlers and children, their mothers change the way in which they speak to them. The changes reflect the mother's recognition of her child's developing understanding of language and then of his attempts to speak. The earliest speech from mothers to babies uses a wide range of intonation and is emotional in content. It uses rhetorical questions and attributes moods and feelings to the baby. The baby himself and his state and features constitute the dominant theme and the tone is one of great warmth. As the baby grows older, the content of the mother's speech changes to reflect and extend his interest in his environment. Comments on objects and activities that are immediately apparent take the place of comments on the child's moods and feelings. These changes in 'mother-talk' occur when the baby is around 3–4 months old. During the first few months, parents start to be aware of the infant's attention to speech and perceive the beginning of comprehension or word recognition. This leads them to use more naming and repetition.

As the infant starts to produce words, the mother responds in such a way as to affirm his attempts and encourage him to continue. The parents perceive the child's use of words as a further sign of his understanding of language and so continue to use language as a means, not only of stimulating and encouraging him but of controlling his behaviour. The Bristol study (Wells, 1985) showed that parents relied upon language to control children as young as 15 months. The directives tended to be short and simple but used the normal adult grammar. The use of speech for control purposes is, of course, unlikely to be effective unless supported by physical action. Unless a child associates the removal of an object with an injunction against banging it, kicking it, throwing it down etc., then spoken injunctions are unlikely to restrain him. This simple example immediately throws up the impossibility of disassociating spoken language from all the complexities of the child–mother relationship and of its individual nature.

Lieven (1982) discusses the characteristics of speech to children to emphasise the importance of individual variation. For example, Lieven, Pine and Dresner Barnes (1992), describe how different routes in language development can be more productive than they might appear. They describe how 'frozen phrases', item-learnt in infancy, can provide in some children, but not all, 'an alternative route into multiword speech'. The implications of this is that there is a need for a degree of flexibility in what might be expected of a child's output at a given age. The consideration of styles of language learning, and the implications of this for early dyadic intervention, have barely been touched upon in the speech and language therapy literature.

Crystal (1986), in a text for parents, illustrates most aptly how research into child language can inform lay people. Teachers and clinicians who take unto themselves the task of advising parents have to try to retain and abstract what is 'good practice' from the revised ideas and current enthusiasms of the research field. The following points may be made when giving instruction to caregivers on how to assist language development in very young children. They have already been well tested and are likely to be durable. The age limits are, of course, approximations.

The first 3 months

Talk to your baby during the periods of physical caring and cuddling. Use natural warm loving tones, playful tones, crooning as your feelings dictate. Respond to your baby's cooing sounds by imitating him or by showing pleasure, smiling and listening. Encourage his sound play by imitating his sounds and adding a few variations of your own. Comment on his looks and behaviour and interpret them aloud.

From 3 to 6 months

Look for different responses to angry and soothing, familiar and unfamiliar voices. Vary the volume and tones of your voice in order to draw your baby's attention to different objects. Make use of all caring routines like bathing and nappy-changing to tell your baby what is going on. Enjoy the responses, smiling, vocalising. Start simple play routines using parts of the body ('This little piggy went to market', 'Walkie round the garden, like a teddy bear', etc.). Start showing simple outline picture books and speaking about what you see.

From 6 to 9 months

Draw baby's attention to common household sounds and voices. Ask questions like 'Where's daddy?', Where's pussy?' and supply answers. 'Here he is'. Play 'Peekaboo'. Use books and toys to interest the baby in names: 'Here's a big car', 'Look at the funny dog'. Respond to baby's communicative signals, shrieks, pointing, bouncing up and down and interpret the signals in words 'You want your milk?', 'You don't like that hat', 'Yes, we're going to go out now'. He may like to joggle about while you sing.

From 9 to 12 months

Talk about things that are happening every day. Use simple, clear speech and make use of routines in order to establish the connection between language and events. Follow the infant's lead. If he indicates something, talk about that. If he is not interested in a book or toy, don't push it but talk about something else. Listen to his attempts to speak and try to interpret them within the context of what you are both doing. Encourage and enjoy but don't demand imitation of your speech. Give the infant plenty of time to respond to your speech and don't carry on a continuous monologue. He will have his own thoughts.

The overall theme is that of interaction and communication. During the first year the mother introduces the baby to ways in which he can participate in and then control his environment. She does this from a basis of consistent, loving nurture. Prevention of delay at this level lies in the promotion of interaction, not the specific reinforcement of training of any single pre-speech skill. By the end of the first year the infant should be capable of recognising words and phrases that reoccur frequently in his daily life. His own utterances may be of a number of types and this will affect the way in which his parents attempt to encourage him. First, they will adapt their language to the level at which they perceive the child comprehends. Secondly, they will respond to the kind of utterance the child uses.

The process of language discovery by the child, assisted by the parent, is both highly pleasurable and non-didactic. The process is not one that proceeds through attention to language rules but through the pleasure of each participant in the behaviour of the other. Those who really enjoy the discovery of language can use it to build skills and interests that will be of permanent benefit to the child. The extension of the process in this way is beautifully illustrated in Dorothy Butler's delightful treatise *Babies Need Books* (Butler, 1988). Butler starts by attempting to interest babies in books when they are a few months old. A book that has bright, simple outlines on a white page will attract the baby's attention if he is shown it at a propitious time, i.e. when alert but not tired, fretful, hungry or wet. Butler points out that the business of holding the baby and directing his attention to the picture is pleasurable for both parties so the experience will not be a total loss, even if the child responds little. Butler develops her thesis by making very practical, concrete suggestions as to the best books to use at different ages.

Such a practice as regular reading to the child is one that can be thoroughly recommended to all parents but it does need to be practically followed up. If people are not used to having books around the home, they will need to be told what to find and how to find it. They will need directing towards infant book and toy libraries and then towards public libraries. It must be explained to parents who are not themselves readers that books offer the infant a much richer experience than does the over-stimulating television screen. This may have a place later on but not for the very young child who needs to identify a few things over and over again in circumstances of quiet caring. As parents start to use simple books they will become more interested in seeking out others. The tele-vision screen does not allow selection or participation in this way.

The early use of books to give pleasure and stimulate interest in language is a far cry from the techniques which are designed to turn infants into prodigies. These have no place in this text. An infant who has learned early in life that books are attractive objects will have a constant source of language nourishment. Not only his parents but all visiting adults may be pressed into reading to him or talking about pictures. He will soon learn to name the pictures and memorise short passages and so can display his own skill in 'reading aloud'. This will naturally encourage him to master reading and his developing language skills will increase the likelihood of his doing so.

Sharing a book with a young child is also very enjoyable for the adult. Not only does it provide a less exhausting form of entertainment than most but it allows for early conversation that a lack of intelligibility on the one side and resourcefulness on the other might otherwise preclude. If two people are looking at a picture and one makes some kind of noise, it is easy for the other to say 'Yes, it is a dog, a big black dog', etc. This 'shared focus' is one of the aspects of motherese, and one that has led to its promotion as a teaching technique (see also White-hurst et al., 1988, on accelerating language development through picture book reading).

The focus of intervention with young children with speech and language delays is now almost entirely prevention based. Muir (1992) reports on the progress of one initiative for parent workshops as a forum for giving information to carers. The emphasis in such workshops is to imbue in parents the confidence to take part in the process of helping their child. Feedback from parents after the course indicated that giving information and training to carers can alleviate anxiety about the child's development, but that intensive courses may also improve knowledge and provide a more cost-effective service.

Prevention by intervention

The first year

Interest in associating 'mother-talk' with the earliest stages of the mother–child relationship is now sufficiently strong to prompt early intervention. An example can be found in Boston, USA where a number of steps were taken to help mothers from disadvantaged and disturbed backgrounds in interacting with their babies. The babies were born to mothers who were not prepared for them and did not know how to manage them. Some were teenagers, many were single parents, many had histories of disturbed or antisocial behaviour. It was hoped that by promoting the skills of parenting, professionals might be able to encourage a more hopeful and positive outlook in the mothers. The speech-language pathologist's contribution to the programme was presented at the American Speech-Language-Hearing Association convention (Proctor, 1982). The mothers were shown how to incorporate loving, warm-toned speech into their caring routines. Wide-ranging intonation, cooing, singing and other gentle, expressive vocalisations were used by the speech-language pathologists and the mothers were asked to imitate. The object was to start a communicative, loving interaction through voice that could be easily perpetuated and developed as the baby responded.

The idea is certainly an appealing one but it needs to be propagated with great care. If mothers are feeling angry, bewildered, frightened or helpless, the attempt to teach them to speak in warm soothing tones will be at best useless and at worst harmful. The infant may very well be frightened and confused by the mixed messages coming from sentimental words with an underlay of hostility and soothing tones with an edge of fear. Counselling and practical help with social needs and personal problems must precede or at least accompany guidance on how to change language behaviour.

There are prophylactic measures to help unresponsive babies and those at risk for language delay, which are simply attempts to give normal experience in a heightened way. Such measures may be found in a number of texts on early communication (e.g. Coupe and Goldbart, 1987; Warner, 1987).

When the infant is at risk for profound handicap, early efforts may be concentrated on showing him how he can affect his environment. Parents and caregivers are advised how to make their responses contingent upon the infant's attempts to move, vocalise or look. Not only does the infant gain pleasure from the response but he starts to realise that activity is productive. He learns that what he does makes a difference to what happens to him. In order to increase an infant's awareness of the importance of language, we must help him first to make sense of what he hears.

Auditory stimulation

All babies benefit from help in listening selectively to environmental sounds because these are now so many and varied that their total impact can be overwhelming. Parents may need guidance with babies who are unresponsive to sound and babies who are distressed by sound may indicate real problems in auditory perception and processing as well as in acuity. Demonstration should be given of how to attract the infant's interest towards a soundmaker by first making it a focus of visual interest. When the noise is produced, the object is well in view and the noise can be repeated. Many parents make the mistake of trying to test a child's reactions to sound by making noises behind his back or when he is engrossed in some activity. Such tactics may achieve a once only response if the sound is loud but they are not part of auditory training. The training consists of building up associations between sounds and objects and activities. If the infant is unresponsive, the mother may be shown how to heighten interest by using an attractive toy with a squeaker, or by rattling a brightly coloured box with something inside, opening the box, taking the object out, putting it back and rattling it again. Caregivers should be advised to show infants the sources of sound by carrying them to the window when the cars are hooting, tracking down the telephone when it rings, listening as well as looking when the television is turned on. Then the range of sounds should be increased: the sound of paper being torn or crumpled, sugar being sifted, tea being stirred.

Children who are not able to attach meaning to sounds will start to ignore them. In some cases this can lead to profound inhibition and withdrawal (Ward, 1984). If this seems to be the case, carefully graded auditory stimulation should be given by professionals in the parents' presence to make sure that everyone knows the limit of the child's tolerance. If babies show excessive sensitivity to sounds, parents should be encouraged to persist in reducing fear. When household objects are being used that generate sudden noise (and there are a great many of these), the infant should, where possible, be prepared. The object should be within his sight and the parent should say 'Here it is, it's going to make a noise' then generate the noise for a short while and then switch the machine off and comment again. The object with all controlled auditory stimulation is to keep the child aware of sounds as being potentially meaningful without letting him become overwhelmed and distressed by them. The stimulation may thus involve capitalising upon the normal and inevitable noises of the household. It should also include quiet times when small sounds and quiet music may be enjoyed and books may be read.

The notion of prevention by early intervention has been brought sharply into focus by the work of Ward (1996). Ward and her colleagues carried out a study of the effects of intervention at a very early stage with a large number of language-delayed children. These children had been detected primarily because of abnormal auditory attention behaviours in infancy. The outcome of a very small amount of intervention was startling: children with early language delays improved rapidly to normal with only a few hours of intervention based solely on input. Ward points out that when followed up at a later age there was not one language-impaired child in the cohort (of over 100) and suggests tentatively that early auditory stimulation may be the key to prevention of confirmed developmental language disorders (an observation that may have a connection with the work of Tallal).

Sound production

As well as responding to environmental sounds and to the speech of others, the infant needs to enjoy the sounds he can produce himself. He first learns the effect of his sounds on others by parental response to his crying. If he is to move on to master the complexities of a speech–sound system as a vehicle for communication, he must get some satisfaction from his early attempts. He is able to demonstrate to others that he is physically capable of generating streams of sound well before he is expected to use speech. If he fails to demonstrate this, there will be concern about his potential for spoken language. Thus the babbling period of babyhood is extremely important because the infant receives pleasure and reinforcement in speech–sound production and the parents are reassured about his speech productive ability. The phenomenon of babbling will therefore be considered in some detail.

Babbling

A relationship has long been posited between the babble sounds that infants make and the words that they subsequently speak. This putative relationship has been explored by different groups of professionals including those interested in a systematic phonology (Locke, 1983), those interested in the manner in which learning operates upon sound production (Winitz, 1969) and those concerned with abnormalities of utterance as a means of identifying handicap (Rutter, Bartak and Newman, 1971; Byers Brown, Bendersky and Chapman, 1986; Rutter, 1987). Rutter has drawn attention to babbling as a significant factor in language disorder by including it in his guidelines for the identification of such disorders (Rutter, 1987):

'A disorder may be suspected .... if babble has been reduced or unusual in quality'.

The identification of such babble is, however, no simple matter. Many studies of babbling that is abnormal have been carried out from recordings of infants known to be at risk (Oller, 1980; Grunwell and Russell, 1987). Moreover, the recordings must in some cases be subjected to instrumental analysis before the normality or abnormality of the babbling can be determined. This is a far cry from requiring parents to identify 'unusual' babble patterns in their own homes. Byers Brown, Bendersky and Chapman (1986) demonstrated that medical personnel can be trained to distinguish between different kinds of babbling activity and thereby to gain some estimate of the infant's speech–sound age. To do this, though, demands both time and practice. Information about the quality of infant babble is likely to be unreliable therefore. However, information about the timing may be more useful.

Babbling is primarily associated with movement. Kent (1984) suggests that reduplicated babbling is not a limited phonological process but rather a developmental process in which cyclicity is used to motor advantage. This places babbling within a developmental framework in which language and a motor system co-emerge. Stark (1981) previously pointed out that babbling first occurs in the context of playing with objects rather than when interacting with another person. Van der Stelt and Koopmans van Beinum (1986) discussed the significance of babbling within a hierarchical order of motor functioning. If the late babble is one of a series of late emerging motor functions it obviously prompts investigation as part of those functions.

Speech and language therapists are familiar with the lack of babbling reported not only by parents of cerebral palsied children but also by parents of children who turn out to be severely apraxic. In the case of cerebral palsy, work is started with babies as part of a whole neuro-developmental therapy. Oral movements are stimulated by tactile and kinaesthetic means to promote a number of activities: feeding, kissing, babbling and speech.

Babbling has been a feature of other developmental therapies but here its role is less clear. Certainly it provides a highly pleasurable activity for child and therapist, if the child is very young and the therapist very enthusiastic. Recent research into the number of different strategies used by early speakers suggests that it may not always be the best procedure. Apraxic children have not necessarily been able to bridge the gap between babbling movements and the organised sequence required for speech.

When infants are reported to lack variety in their speech–sound production, and to be delayed in gross and fine motor skills, these functions may certainly be stimulated and encouraged together. Rhythmic sound play, singing and clapping games, action games with the child supplying a sound at the end of the sequence are all useful and pleasurable ways of helping movement. They heighten the excitement and hence the activity level that may enable the child to be more productive. However, it may still be important to encourage the use of a communicative strategy consisting of vowels only. If the parent responds to such signals, the child feels success. Moreover, the child may receive the linguistic advantages of contingent maternal speech, shared topic, extension, etc without excessive demands being placed upon his motor skills.

Babbling has been shown to have a place in the assessment of emerging language as a feature of cognition, as a feature of cognitive delay and autism. The babbling itself does not demand intervention though it may point the way to other forms of intervention (Wetherby et al., 1986; Del Priore, Valance and Day, 1987). Babbling is also of major interest to phonologists who look to it for first evidence of systematic sound production as a forerunner to phonology. Locke (1983, 1986) has reviewed this subject extensively. Failure to develop a systematic phonology cannot be prevented, however, by intervention at the babbling stage. We might possibly be able to expand the infant's babbling repertoire, if the family tendencies were suggestive of phono-logical disability. But the phonology could only be developed as words were acquired, which involves another organisational level.

In summary, babbling shows evidence of motor coordination and subsequently of auditory and cognitive alertness. Its absence attracts attention to those areas. Encouraging babbling will not work any mira-cles but it may give the infant a little push along the developmental path. Any increase of skill opens up possibilities. It indicates responsiveness and evidence of ability to learn. When children are developmentally delayed, all such evidence is important. It will be significant whether the increase in babbling comes about as the result of promoting another type of activity (crawling, object play) or as the result of auditory and linguistic stimulation and interaction.

Speech and language therapists tend to believe that there is a strong association between lack of babble and subsequent speech disorders. However, as has been pointed out previously, speech and language ther-apists have access to a special sample only. There is some research support for the contention that all normal infants babble at some point (Van der Stelt and Koopmans van Beinum, 1986). They also coo, laugh, vocalise to smiling adults, use vowel glides and indicate communicative intent. Whilst babble is likely to continue to attract the research field, it should not completely dominate the prophylactic one. Mothers have been known to become very anxious as to whether or not their babies are babbling 'properly'. This does no good to them or to their relation-ship with their infant. If babies are to be stimulated to babble as part of a guidance programme, it must be done in a relaxed and happy manner.

Babbling stimulation

A vital component of any stimulation programme is knowing when to stimulate. Because the generation of a babble demands coordinated activity of breathing, vocalisation and movement of the articulators, it cannot be expected from a very immature mechanism. The literature does not yield cases of repetitive babbling during the first 2 months of life, even in the most advanced babies. We must therefore assume that a number of other activities must take place first. This is why the emphasis in neuro-developmental therapy is upon a gradual progression from one skill to another. The time to stimulate babbling occurs after the oral reflexes of rooting, sucking and biting have started to wane. The tongue is thus more capable of moving independently. The infant's respiratory health must be such that he is not struggling for breath or breathing so quickly and shallowly that a string of babble sounds cannot be supported. Once an infant has achieved such a string of sounds, he will essay another, even if he has quite severe respiratory congestion. Noisy breathing sounds are distressing but do not necessarily prevent babble from emerging. Nevertheless, it is unwise to use tactile and kinaesthetic stimulation in such cases. The adult should rely upon auditory stimulation, smiling, and an enthusiastic response. If the babble chains occur when the infant is apart from the adult, he should not be interrupted.

Mothers may be encouraged by experienced speech and language therapists to move the baby's lips and jaw while he is vocalising in order to give him the sensation of what normal movement is like. When such training is given, it is generally in conjunction with a programme of physical therapy. Such training must only take place with careful demonstration and with reference to the one child. If general advice is given, it is wisest to restrict it to such measures as the following:

- Extend the infant's overall desire to move by placing attractive objects so as to encourage head turning, rolling and general pursuit.
- Promote hand and hand-to-mouth activities by giving the infant different objects to hold and to take to his mouth; objects should be such that they cannot be drawn in and swallowed.
- Use sound play with the infant, either by initiating it during phases of lively interaction or by echoing his brief babble attempts.
- Extend the range of babble sounds, e.g. after a number of 'dadada' chains, try 'bababa', use repetitive consonant–vowel chains until the range is extended and then use combinations 'dadaba' 'bagaga'; vary the stress and volume.
- As babble appears, stimulate general listening skills so that the auditory–motor loop may be strengthened; try to incorporate turntaking into babble practice.
- The final injunction is more difficult to convey. Briefly, it is 'do not confuse a thinking baby'. In babbling, as in all skills, the baby may start coming to certain conclusions. He may like the sound he has just made and want to try it again, or he may have made some discovery from it which prompts him to try something else. Everyone concerned with the child should try to understand his own temperament and way of going about things.

Sound imitation

There is general agreement that some children are better mimics or natural imitators than others and this skill is almost certainly helpful in acquiring phonological patterns. The point became masked early in the study of child language acquisition because it was important to establish that language was not learned by imitation but by making deductions from available data. While we do not learn language through imitation, spoken language is facilitated by practice and here imitation has a role to play. Imitation and role learning can improve phonological memory. Thus, repetition of sound patterns, rhymes and even nonsense words may assist the young child to memorise sound sequences at a later stage. Short-term phonological memory is suggested (Gathercole and Baddeley, 1989), as being associated with development of vocabulary. We are therefore justified in advising mothers to teach children new words through imitation and before this stage to encourage imitation and mimicry of sound patterns. Both immediate and delayed repetition may be employed. While language-delayed children may be slow to acquire words because they lack an overall matrix to support them, others may be slow because of poor phonological skills associated with inability to repeat. Repetition practice at an early age is only likely to do harm if carried out over-zealously and humourlessly. Otherwise it may well be generally useful.

Individual variation in language development

By the end of the first year, the infant is already starting to show some individual characteristics or stylistic preferences in speech. This appears to reflect his own disposition rather than that of his family because different siblings show different preferences. Byers Brown and Lewis (1984); and Byers Brown, (1988) looked at 50 1-year-olds (25 male and 25 female) and found the following: during 25 minutes of child–mother interaction the infant's number of utterances ranged from 99 to 1. As well as showing great variation in quantity, there was variation in kind. The most prolific speakers used both variegated and non-variegated babble, vowels with intonation (melodic cadences), vowels in a sequence with or without glottal stop, vocables and words. A positive correlation was found between an overall factor of productive language range and a factor of productive language competence at 2 years of age. This competence factor was derived from the number of connected utterances used by the child, the mean length of these utterances and the ability to use speech to ask questions, generate information and maintain sociability. The authors concluded that the ability to generate a range of utterances at 1 year was a good predictive sign.

A second group of children showed preference for vowel use and relied strongly on the vowel sequence for communication. There was no overall indication to suggest that their language was delayed at 2 years. Some were advanced, some average, some below average. The authors suggested that this vowel preference was a strategy that might be adopted by the less motorically advanced children in that it maintained communication without demanding fine motor control. The vowel sequences /uh uh uh uh/ were often used with a degree of urgency that demanded a communicative response. Children who used babble and melodic cadence might use them with or without seeming to desire the attention of the mother. These strategies were both expressive of mood and useful in conveying mood and information (not always interpretable by the adult!). The vowel sequence was only used communicatively and thus could be associated with children who were not highly expressive overall.

A third group of 1-year-olds tended to rely upon simple consonant–vowel combinations uttered somewhat explosively—'da'. They did not generate long utterances. A positive correlation was found between this factor of consonant use and a factor of unintelligible (or inadequate) utterance at 2 years. A negative correlation was found between the factor of productive language competence at 2 years. The authors suggested that the consonant use strategy was one employed by the least able communicators, or perhaps by those least interested in communication.

Implications for prevention

Because the children taking part in the above study were only recorded with their mothers at 1 year and then at 2 years, it is not possible to speak about the influence either of the mother's speech or of her behaviour. What the study does illustrate is the strategic choice available and the possibilities of a mismatch of style and temperament between mother and child. Some mothers were equally responsive to a 1-year-old using grunts, points and vowel sequences as to the 2-year-old using words. One could opine that this responsiveness was a factor in the child's progress. Other mothers noticeably communicated much less with their 1-year-olds than with their 2-year-olds. Where the child was strongly expressive and communicative himself, this did not seem to deter him. The combination of an uncommunicative, unexpressive child and an unresponsive mother, though very understandable, was not very propitious.

We can only speculate on the possible effects of interaction when the child is inexpressive and uncommunicative and the mother is highly expressive. In one mother–child dyad observed by Byers Brown and Lewis, the mother talked continuously to her unresponsive, inattentive 1-year-old. He produced his only continuous utterance, a repetitive babble chain, while his mother was briefly out of the room. At 2 years of age the child was non-communicative and the mother unable to engage him. Whose behaviour was the most responsible? Just as such paediatricians as Brazelton gave mothers enormous relief by telling them that they had difficult babies, or that they would have done a fine job with a baby of a different temperament, so speech and language therapists may make the same kind of observations to mothers of speech-delayed children. The mother, as the more skilled partner, has the onus on her to promote language development in the child. However, some mothers have a much easier time than others. When recommending texts to mothers who want to know more about the process, choose those in which information is blended with humour and affection (Crystal, 1986; Butler, 1988) so that rigidity is discouraged.

The second year

If mother and child have arrived at the child's first birthday with confidence in each other as communicators, the way is well prepared for the next phase. As the first words start to appear it will be easier for parents to support and extend language. The ensuing years that see the transition from non-linguistic to linguistic communication will be dominated by the child's struggle to convey meaning. This will involve the negotiation of failed messages (Golinkoff, 1983). The solving of phonological problems and the achievement of early grammar are stimulated by the need to convey meaning to someone who does not have immediate, total comprehension of what you are about. The child also needs to acquire vocabulary to suit his expanding world.

Crystal (1986) and Rescorla (1984) have indicated the categories of words that young children use. The enormous amount of physical activity in which they indulge stimulates interest in action words. Their physical needs and preferences lead to rapid learning of names for different foods, clothing and parts of the body. Their individual environments will prompt the need for animal names, names of friends and relatives and names for different kinds of vehicles. Words signifying location, specificity, description and possession will emerge as soon as the child starts to combine words. Given that the child has normal abilities, good relationships and plenty of things to see and do, there is little need for advice on how to promote language. The child will dictate and the parents respond, elaborate, extend, support and puzzle out his meaning. It is only when something is lacking in the child or in the language support system that advice on how to nourish and stimulate language must be given.

Guidelines for prevention in the second year

Language guidance will try to put the mother and child in touch with each other in order that the kind of interaction and communication that take place normally can be established. The clinician, states Sparks (1989), should help the care-giver to understand why the child is behaving the way he is, and help them to recognise the child's attempt at communication and to understand that any form of communication must be responded to. Advisers will try to dissuade parents from thinking about chronological age and the arbitrary standards this dictates, and draw attention to the child's developmental level. Language cannot emerge until prelinguistic communication has taken place. The play rituals and simple auditory stimulation suitable to early infancy may be demonstrated and advocated. Intervention should concentrate as much on the parent–child interaction as on the behaviour of the child. Subsequent advice will make use of tactics derived from 'motherese':

- Establish a joint focus.
- Let the child determine this focus.
- Use simple, lively language to identify, describe and comment.
- Use questions and supply answers until the child is able to respond.
- Be sensitive to the child's signals both of response and of intention.
- Respond immediately to communicative signals.
- As the child becomes more adept at signalling, make the response contingent upon certain standards, e.g. if words are attempted, reward the attempt; later you may hold out until the approximation is clearer.
- Adapt your speech to the child's developing level of comprehension.
- Elaborate, extend and support the child's statement to affirm its meaning.
- Recast statements in a slightly different form in order to accelerate learning.

The important points to convey are that all situations can be used for language development and that language emerges from context. There is no need to discuss the theory of language development if mothers are happy to accept demonstrations and become successful in finding ways of their own. If mothers or care-givers wish for more information, it can be provided. Weistuch and Byers Brown (1987) report upon a programme of language facilitation in which different groups of mothers were involved. One group of mothers whose children were language-delayed preferred not to explore the literature because they were upset by comparisons between their own children and children who learned language more quickly and easily. Other groups welcomed reading material because it stimulated them to question and to discuss the procedures and to find their own solutions.

The third year

The third year is the one in which language delay may first show itself in a decisive manner and the one in which language disorder may be heralded. Rutter's guidance list starts by saying that children not using simple words by 24 months and/or not using phrases by 33 months need systematic investigation. This is in accord with the findings and opinions of a number of workers (see Chapter 2). Snyder-McClean and McClean (1987) writing about early intervention say that the diagnosis of language delay is not generally made until the child reaches the age at which at least some language production is normally expected – at least 2 years. These authors also say that the diagnosis is made on the basis of discrepancy between overall level of language development and overall level of cognitive or mental development. By contrast, language disability or language disorder are terms only applied to children who have reached a level of development characterised by the production of multi-word utterances, in other words children above the age of 3 years and who manifest very specific discrepancies within their overall linguistic performance level. There is some relationship here to another of Rutter's guidelines: attention should be paid to the course of language development. Once the child has started to use words, is progress moving rapidly ahead on all fronts or is the speed of acquisition less than it should be?

The third year is the one that is probably the most significant from the prophylactic aspect because it gives us the chance to advise about delays and observe development within the framework of advice and support. How should this best be done?

Cooper, Moodley and Reynell (1978) in their well known text on *Helping Language Development* offer a developmental approach that they consider suitable for children between the ages of 2 and 4 years although it can be used for slightly older children. A major tenet is the creation of a language environment for the child. Consequently, parents figure prominently and are indeed integral to the programmes. Warner, Byers Brown and McCartney (1984) give examples of how to work with the child, or the child and parent on an individual basis. Bath (1981) describes an approach to assessment and remediation carried out through the cooperation of the staff of day nurseries. Weistuch and Byers Brown (1987) offer a study showing how mothers were encouraged to assist their children's language development by modifying their own. This therapy through 'motherese' is considered suitable as a single method or one that could be combined with other forms of therapy such as the overall developmental stimulation given in the US Early Intervention/Infant Stimulation Programs.

Early intervention programmes

Currently, educational programmes and related services are available throughout the USA through a combination of federal and state funding. A major piece of legislature was the passing of Public Law 94-142, the Education for all Handicapped Children Act. A subsequent amendment

(1986) has extended provision to cover infants and toddlers as well as preschool children. Because those who work with very young children are continuously being challenged to demonstrate their effectiveness, it is heartening to read the first two items of the 1986 revision.

PL 99-457:

Sec. 671 (a) Findings–the congress finds that there is an urgent and substantial need

1. to enhance the development of handicapped infants and toddlers and to minimize their potential for developmental delay,
2. to reduce the educational costs to our society, including our nation's schools, by minimizing the need for special education and related services after handicapped infants and toddlers reach school age.

Because the demands for accountability in the USA are extremely high, these items indicate the very real effectiveness of early intervention for children with or at risk for developmental disabilities. The programmes supported by this legislation are available for the young handicapped. In order to qualify for admission there must be demonstrable delay in at least two areas: cognitive, motor sensory, socio–emotional and communication/language. Children with speech delay only, would not qualify, nor would the programme be suitable. Indeed, some mothers refuse to enrol their children in the programmes when their main complaint is language delay because they do not want the term 'handicapped' to be attached to them. Children admitted to these programmes receive the attention of an interdisciplinary team and the emphasis is upon assisting all aspects of development. Thus the children are assessed by the whole team and developmental profiles interpretable to professionals and parents are drawn up. Parents are involved at all stages because a declared aim of the early intervention movement is to assist parents in responding to the needs of their developmentally handicapped children and to be sensitive to the changing nature of these needs (see Guralnick and Bennett (1987) for full discussion of the aims and achievements of the early intervention programmes).

Much of the philosophy and many of the procedures of the American early intervention programmes will be familiar to British workers. Working with the parents of handicapped children has been a well recognised sphere of professional activity since the early 1960s and of course in individual circumstances, long before. Speech and language therapists have been very much influenced by such writers and teachers as Dorothy Jeffree and Roy McConkey. However, there is a distinctive national difference in that the American emphasis is upon intervention for all children at risk regardless of what that risk is. Thus within the same programme one might encounter children with cognitive delays, motor impairments, language/communication delays, autism and sensory impairments of hearing and vision. Whilst each child will receive an individual assessment and programme, these will be carried out within the group structure and administered by interdisciplinary or, indeed, transdisciplinary teams.

One advantage of exposing the child to a number of highly trained professionals is that his development will be very closely observed. One would therefore expect that the language-disordered child would start to become evident. According to Rutter's guidelines, the child at risk for language disorder would be well placed within such a multidisciplinary establishment because, in addition to the language features he may display unusual or deviant motor development, socio-emotional or behavioural problems and associated medical problems. It is obviously extremely desirable for mothers that their children should receive treatment in one place and from a team of specialists each member of which is highly conversant with the methods and opinions of the others. Nevertheless objections can be made. Not all children need such a concentration of expertise, and it is, of course, very expensive. In choosing a number of activities to suit all children there is very real danger of coming up with some that suit none of them. It is very difficult to keep up with the research and activities pertinent to any particular area when working all the time in a transdisciplinary capacity. Like all good endeavours, the Early Intervention Program may be saluted by those working in other settings without the compulsion to adopt it. The UK has managed to achieve some excellent results through a combination of early therapy and special nursery placement. The NHS allows infants to receive this therapy at any age. In view of the individual variation in language development, it is very fitting that different approaches be attempted. However, in view of the similarities in their needs, it is essential that all such approaches involve the parents or care-givers.

The Position paper on the role and responsibility of speech and language therapists in child language disability (College of Speech Therapists, 1988a) makes the following provisions:

* When language development predominantly complements an overall developmental delay, the speech and language therapist may monitor progress on a review basis to ensure that appropriate development continues and prevent problems arising for a child who is known to be at risk.
* When receptive and/or expressive language development is significantly delayed in relation to other skill areas, the speech and language therapist is more actively involved and may provide appropriate materials/programmes for parents and teachers to use with the child; progress should be monitored regularly by the speech and language therapist; and periods of regular therapy may be indicated.

- When the aetiological factor is pervasive, it may conceal a language disability or prevent the development of communication; the speech and language therapist will monitor progress in order to form a diagnosis and decide on appropriate intervention, as for example in some cases of learning disorder or profound mental handicap.

It is important to remember that this is quoted from a position paper and not from a text on how to work with language-delayed or disordered children. Nevertheless some points may be made in relation to monitoring. It is only too easy for monitoring to become periodic assessment where the therapist carries out tests and ask questions of the parent and then provides information as to whether or not the child has progressed. To monitor is to keep a watch over. It should involve thorough discussion with the parents who may be asked to keep diaries, recordings or vocabulary lists. It involves the demonstration of ways in which language can be stimulated and suggestions as to the best times and places in which to do this. It should recommend all the normal activities through which language can be enriched at the developmental level of the child. Sometimes the parent and therapist may experiment with some material that is not immediately obvious and keep records of reactions. An interesting example of the response of a handicapped child to unusual language stimulation can be seen in Dorothy Butler's second book *Cushla and Her Books* (1987). Butler recounts the way in which a book-based compensatory programme was used for her grandchild who was developmentally handicapped. The outstanding feature of this text is in showing how something of a profound importance to a family, namely reading, could be used to assist the integration and development of a child who might have been deemed unable to participate. The interest in books is central to the whole family and so uniquely useful as a language teaching method.

During the process of monitoring, the therapist may be able to find out about the interests of the family and suggest ways in which these can be shared with the child in such a way as to extend primitive language skills. The child's response will give further clues upon which the next phase of activity may be based. This early prophylactic period is thus one in which the whole family may be prepared for long-term help and the therapist may find out what kind of help is likely to be needed. When a more thorough assessment of language skills is subsequently carried out, the parents will have been fully prepared for it and so will the child.

Some indication of the positive effects of this kind of language monitoring upon the family of the language-delayed child is given in the following account. The child in question was developmentally delayed and unresponsive with the most severe aspect of the delay being language and communication. He subsequently showed evidence of semantic–pragmatic language disorder with good powers of repetition but difficulties in comprehension and word meaning. His mother writes:

> These visits [to the language clinic] were a source of enjoyment to J but to me
> they were much more. These sessions were like an infusion of energy and
> hope for the future. Each week we had something positive and concrete to
> work on at home. Life became more structured. These were times of fun and
> noise and great enthusiasm. I sometimes think that I benefited even more
> than J did for here I met with a positive and optimistic attitude which was just
> the remedy for the despondency I had experienced during the last 18
> months. These precious hours were morale boosters, and probably one of
> the most important factors in helping the family recover from what had
> seemed to be a major disaster.

At this stage of prevention, the therapist is concerned, above all, to
help the family to come together and to find confidence through interaction. The discovery that a child may be handicapped is shocking and
when the long-term consequences are not predictable no one knows
how to behave. Prevention operates to reduce abnormal interactions
that come about through anxiety and doubt. This in turn allows the
normal human resourcefulness to come into being and members of the
family start coming up with helpful activities. In talking about this kind
of prevention, we are recognising that a comprehensive assessment of
the language-delayed child's abilities and deficits may not have taken
place and the measures advocated prepare everyone for this assessment.
Following it, the process of tertiary prevention may be started. This will
be discussed in our text following the chapter on assessment and chapters dealing more specifically with the nature of language disorders.

Older children

Work with the school-aged child is likely to be remedial rather than
prophylactic except in so much as intervention at one level may reduce
complications later on. It may facilitate another level of language
learning. In a text devoted to written language difficulties Snowling
(1985a) and Bryant (1985) pose questions about prevention. Indeed,
Bryant asks the rather simple and basic question as to whether or not
steps can be taken before the vulnerable child starts school, which will
allow him to pick up skills that are necessary to avoid becoming a
dyslexic. Bryant refers to the experimental studies, case histories and
epidemiological surveys that have been carried out to enrich our knowledge and notes that no-one has posed the question: How can we stop
the problem in the first place? Bryant reviews evidence to support or
negate the idea that dyslexic children form a group that is qualitatively
different from other children. He comes down in favour of the
continuum of reading ability with the dyslexics at the bottom end. This,

he thinks is encouraging because it implies that what helps everyone will help them 'So we just help them all'. Bryant then suggests that the best way to help them all is to improve the skill with sounds in words. He refers to the wealth of evidence that suggests that this is a skill that can be fostered and enjoyed. He suggests that we encourage our preschool children to listen to nursery rhymes and poems and then to make up their own poems. This is entirely in accord with the advice we would give to assist spoken language. Snowling, in her editorial summing up at the end of the volume, makes it clear that there are opposing views to Bryant's. Nevertheless, she affirms that early intervention and training in sounds is effective even although there may still be a hard core of dyslexics not amenable to such methods.

Locke (1989), writing about the Birmingham schools programme, points out that a large number of children entering school are shown to have poor communication skills. During the primary intervention period, emphasis is placed upon the development of oral language. 'Children promote their own learning through language, talking to themselves and others as they meet new experiences. Talking should be seen as a fundamental way in which children clarify their ideas and solve problems.' This activity may be seen as both prophylactic and diagnostic because it will soon throw up those children who have special communicative needs. As Beveridge and Conti-Ramsden (1987) point out, there will be differences between the degrees of skill children bring to language learning. Differences in children's memory, verbal reasoning abilities, inferential abilities and verbal playfulness are all mentioned as being important. The skilled teacher can do much to encourage all these attributes and thus promote interest and confidence in language learning and in language use.

Chapter 4
The underlying nature of developmental language disorders

HILARY GARDNER

Summary

This chapter begins with an outline of principles of information processing as a basis for understanding complex language mechanisms. It then continues by discussing the possible application of such a model to neurobiological, cognitive and linguistic aspects as a precursor to understanding how impairment or inefficiency of processing may contribute to developmental language disorders.

Language-disordered children appear very different in the patterns of strengths and weaknesses that they display. In recent times a considerable amount of research has helped to identify the subgroups of language disorder and it has become clear that even overtly similar patterns of language functioning may have different underlying deficits. It is essential if we are to come to terms with the entire range of language disorders that we should be able to see them in relation to a theoretical model that may offer cohesion and indicate relationships. This chapter will therefore discuss language disorder within the context of an *information processing model*.

Because each language level is described separately, it would be misleading to deduce that they are discrete. Rather, they represent different facets of the same coin. There are obvious overlaps and interactions between them, for example psycholinguistic theories forming a bridge between cognitive neuropsychology and pure linguistics. The emphasis on the eclectic nature of these models is imperative in order to get a balanced view of the literature, much of which takes an exclusive stance depending on the viewpoint of the writer.

There are two major schools of thought as to the underlying causes of developmental language disorders pertaining to cognition and linguistic functioning. On one side there are those who argue that the disorders are rooted in an overall processing deficit, the effect of which is most clearly manifested in poor language skills. These theories will predominantly be discussed under the 'cognitive' heading, although some researchers straddle the cognitive/linguistic divide by talking of specific deficits in, for instance, auditory phonological processing. On the other hand theorists have struggled to produce a successful computer model of language learning and this has prompted lines of research that search for some specific 'modular' deficit in the innate LAD (learning acquisition device) that infants are purported to possess. Such theories of language disorder will be discussed in the section on 'linguistic' models.

An information processing model

Before a more detailed consideration of specific language models, some preliminary description of the principles of information processing may be beneficial as this provides a framework in which to consider the special place of language.

Essentially, information processing as has been described in Chapter 1 can be reduced to a very simple level in which there are three main components: a receiver, a control system and an effector. The human being as the processor is seen to play an active part, that is to say, they are not passive recipients of incoming information. Stelmach (1982) postulates some important assumptions that underlie information processing.

- First is the fact that there are many stages between the reception of the incoming stimulus and the subsequent response. In fact, the nature of the response may be of minor significance in the processing chain, for it will have been predetermined by the previous stages, although a number of options will have been available.
- Second, the sequence of events is invariable, for each stage can only operate on information received from the previous stimulus. The notion of a control system operating in the absence of a receiver is ludicrous. The ringing of a telephone bell for example, has first to be detected and recognised before being answered, in that order.
- Third, each stage effects change in the information it receives; this is an event that takes time.
- Finally, once processing at a particular stage is complete, the information is made available to the next stage.

A simple model of information processing is given in Figure 4.1. There are two important controlling mechanisms that operate in the form of feedback and feedforward. *Feedback* involves an ongoing monitoring facility as sensory information is fed into the system from the motor activity that is generated. *Feedforward* has an anticipatory function. Thus comparison can be made at each stage between incoming

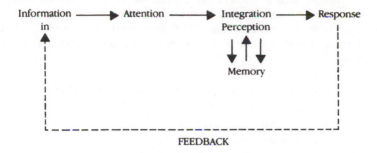

Figure 4.1 Schematic representation of an information processing model.

information and the established pattern so that control is exercised on the response before it becomes overt. Feedforward may therefore be described as an internal monitoring system that has a capability of detecting errors prior to output.

We will now consider some of the human biological correlates of the simple information processing model that are basic prerequisites for normal language development. The pathway from reception to response is described.

Neurobiological aspects of language processing

Language represents a synthesis of psychological, linguistic and physiological behaviours (Edwards, 1984). In this section we consider some aspects of the neurophysical system that underlies language. It is still not understood completely how much language centres are encapsulated from general cognitive function. Recent genetic studies of certain subgroups of SLI children, such as those by Van der Lely and Stollwerck (1996), are providing mounting evidence for a biological, domain specific and modular basis to language. Other identifiable genetically defined physical or metabolic disorders such as Williams' syndrome also demonstrate that language can develop to a level that well exceeds the child's cognitive abilities (Bellugi et al., 1993). Conversely in others, such as Down's syndrome, language abilities can lag well behind.

Cognitive neuropsychology is a discipline that has looked at brain damage and concomitant language breakdown in adults and has been successful in establishing localisation of certain language skills to specific areas of the brain. However, it must be remembered that the language centres of the brain do not map directly on to the information processing models outlined in this chapter.

McCarthy and Warrington (1990) say:

It is sometimes tempting to think of 'box and arrow' models of cognitive function as being an accurate account of encapsulated systems or modules. It is
necessary to bear in mind that models of 'functional architecture'...... are
highly abstract formalisms rather than something 'out there' waiting to be
localised (p. 369).

There are complex inter-relationships between areas of the brain, and
the more diffuse effects of brain damage imply that some caution needs
to be taken when considering localisation theories. Also, caution is
needed in equating the loss of a well-developed system in an adult with
the child's brain where apparent plasticity allows language to develop
despite the loss of supposedly critical sites (even complete hemispherec-
tomy). The medical taxonomies of child language disorder based on the
disabilities found in adult brain damage fail to reflect adequately the
nature of developmental disorders and other frameworks can enhance
the picture (see Chapter 8).

It is, however, worth describing briefly the complexities of the neural
pathways and some developmental factors that are important when we
come to consider alternative explanations of language development and
disorder.

Reception of information

Shallice (1984) points out that simple motor and sensory functions are
the only clearly encapsulated subsystems in information processing
terms. The central nervous system structures governing the reception of
incoming information may be divided into primary and secondary
cortical regions. Taking the auditory system as a starting point, afferent
impulses from the organ of Corti in the inner ear travel via the reticular
system to the primary auditory cortex. Within the reticular system, which
is also concerned with attention, preliminary selection and inhibition of
input takes place. Mysak (1976) describes this lower order receptor
system as having three functions: the orienting of the head to the source
of the signal, stimulating arousal mechanisms and generating efferent
impulses to regulate the responsiveness of the auditory system at any
level. This last function is effected through descending nerve fibres that
provide feedback so that adjustments can be made to the incoming
stimuli at points along the tract in the many relay stations (nuclei).

All ascending fibres of the eighth cranial nerve pass through the thal-
amus and it is thought that further refinement of the signal takes place at
this level. Within the cerebral cortex, Luria (1970) describes three zones
that are essential to auditory perception. This first is the 'primary projection area', which lies deep in the temporal lobe. This part is said to
contain cells that are specifically adapted to respond to certain frequen-

cies of sound. This has led some workers to speculate that early feature discrimination may take place here. Geschwind and Levitsky (1968) first noted that this particular zone is larger in the left (dominant) side than in the right.

The second cortical unit is the 'association temporal cortex', which lies in the superior posterior temporal region (the classic Wernicke's area). Its function is concerned with the refinement, recognition and synthesis of signals that have already received primary analysis in the projection cortex. It is likely that at this point, phonological coding takes place including features of sequence and timing. From this area a pathway runs in the arcuate fasciculus forward to Broca's area, which is the association cortex lying anterior to the motor strip concerned with movement for speech. The association temporal cortex has an important role in relation to episodic memory storage but it is thought that long-term (semantic) memory is stored throughout the brain.

Integration and internal representation

The function of the third unit is that of integration of perceptions from the different modalities into internal representations. Luria calls this region the 'tertiary zone'. Anatomically this lies at the junction of the auditory, visual and somalesthetic association cortices. This has been called 'the association area of association areas'–it is the angular gyrus, occurs only in humans and is one of the later parts of the brain to become myelinated.

Innervation is bilateral for hearing, but experimental evidence derived from many studies usually involving dichotic listening tasks indicates that the dominant hemisphere is the main processor of linguistic input, although, to a lesser extent, the non-dominant hemisphere does participate. Springer and Deutsch (1989) state that the right hemisphere can comprehend sentences at a low level, recognising noun and verb categories equally well but does not process syntax as in the left hemisphere. There is a possibility that a change in this pattern occurs where damage is sustained in infancy, but there is variation expressed in views about the extent to which the assumption of the language role is taken over by the non-dominant hemisphere (see, for example, Woods and Carey, 1979; Murdoch, 1990).

So far in this discussion of the neurophysiology of language we have paralleled the information processing model in relation to input, integration and storage. We now need to consider response, that is to say, how language is actually produced. Between perception and ideation and between ideation–the germ of an idea of what we want to say (according to Lashley, 1951)–and the onset of speech, there are gaps that at the present time remain unbridged. Obviously, before any programming of language can take place, there must be an intention to speak.

Production

Planning of an utterance entails the preparation of schemata that best fit the requirements of the linguistic programme. Such schemata are built up during language development through the integration of the incoming sensory information and these are stored as outlined above. The fundamental goals are thus defined at cortical level, but the coordinative action necessary for speech production is the outcome of multi-level activity within the central nervous system. Important points of control would be at cerebellar, subcortical and brain-stem levels. This hierarchy represents a consensus rather than a central executive mode of control. The subcortical and cerebellar areas are associated with ordering and motivational aspects as well as refining and modifying effects on motor schemata.

Hebb in 1949 proposed a theory of 'motor equivalence' and this was extensively developed by MacNeilage (1970). During the learning of an activity, integrated percepts from auditory, visual and proprioceptive channels are built up to form internalised patterns of that activity. This is not a detailed plan, but an overall schema that is directed towards the target. There is therefore allowance for possible variation in the circumstances in which the target is reached. A good example is that where a person can speak intelligibly whilst a pipe is clutched between the teeth. To achieve this there must be a series of adaptive movements of tongue and lips to allow for the relative immobility of the jaws. A more striking example is the degree of intelligibility achieved by patients following partial glossectomies and this also is the result of compensatory movements designed to meet a target.

Developmental aspects of neurophysiology

There seems to be growing evidence that language acquisition has a marked biological–maturational component (Flavell, Miller and Miller, 1993). Plante (1991) suggests that the identifiable genetic contributions to language disorder may be traced to neuroanatomical differences. Netsell (1986) states that the most sensitive period for acquisition of motor control of speech appears to be between 3 and 12 months and this is also a period of rapid myelination of the nerve tracts. There is a direct relationship between language acquisition and myelination of the higher centres of the central nervous system. Delays during this time, he considers, may have serious implications for the normal development of coordination of movement within the vocal tract. It is during this stage that the fundamental schemata for speech patterns begin to be laid down. Dobbing (1972) describes how the brain grows rapidly from the last 10 weeks of fetal life to about 2 years of age. By the last 13 weeks, the adult number of neurones is present. The subsequent growth spurt, therefore, is concerned with the building up of interneuronal connections. Possible deleterious consequences of interruption of the growth spurt have been discussed in Chapter 2.

How far we are specifically biologically pre-tuned to develop language is a point of debate but there is evidence, even from birth, of left-hemisphere specialisation for language-like stimuli (Prescott and de Caspar, 1990). Evidence also comes from the universally similar patterns of development that occur, whatever mother tongue the child is exposed to. Further evidence also rests with the fact there is an optimal age for language learning as shown by the relative decline in the ability to learn a language after puberty (Johnston and Newport, 1989). This type of evidence is used to support 'nativistic' theories of language development and the assumption of an innate 'language acquisition device' that enables humans to learn the complexities of language. This is especially important in some linguistic theories of language learning as we shall see later.

Any theory of language development and disorder must be able to explain the varied pattern of skills that SLI children can have, for instance their good non-verbal abilities in comparison to their verbal skills, their ability to discriminate words that they cannot produce and so forth. These discrepancies have all variously caused difficulties for the models we are to discuss.

Cognitive bases of language development

The intact neural pathways allow children to perform basic cognitive and perceptual functions basic to the processing of language. These are:

Attention

As human beings we are constantly bombarded with incoming information from the environment–sights, sounds, smells, movement, etc–were we to attempt to attend to all of these, the result would be one of utter confusion. There is a limit to the amount of information the brain can process at any one time. Miller (1967) in his eloquent essay, 'The magical number of 7 plus or minus 2' refers to the information bottleneck that can only be overcome by the organisation of incoming material into manageable sequential chunks or units. This of course is closely related to memory.

Moray (1972) describes a theory of capacity attention that also suggests an overall limit to the amount of information to which the system can attend, regardless of the number of channels involved. This means that up to a capacity point, multimodal attention is possible, but once past that point, there will be a decrement in processing ability. This theory is of interest when one considers the low threshold of multimodal attention in some language-disordered children and this is a crucial factor in cognitive theories of language processing.

Moray's views are in conflict with another major theory of attention, that proposed by Broadbent in 1958. In order to avoid the problem of an overloaded system he suggested that the only way in which information can be handled is sequentially. Earlier stages of detection and recognition, he maintained, can take place without attention so that, peripherally, multichannels can carry information in parallel. In order to process two simultaneous messages, one is transferred to the short-term memory store. The longer it is held there, the greater is its degradation. Obviously there is a strong element of selectivity in such an operation. This will relate to the strength of the stimulus and also the subject's familiarity with it.

Whichever model is favoured, it is accepted that attention plays a crucial part in language acquisition. The development of attention has been described by Kagan (1971) who proposed three stages: the first is that of total attention, which is however, fleeting and that decreases rapidly as the object is removed and interest fades. This would coincide with pre-object permanence in Piagetian terms. The second stage is that which he terms 'discrepancy'; this is when some discordant feature is introduced into the situation and this serves to sharpen attention. The third stage is that of density of stimuli. Here the individual is able to integrate different stimuli to produce novel experiences.

Perception

Language is received through two principal sensory channels: 'auditory' and 'visual'. Spoken language relies mainly on the former although concomitant information is relayed along visual channels through gesture, facial expression, etc. For written language to be understood, an intact visual sensory channel is necessary, although this again may be enhanced through the medium of accompanying auditory stimuli. To a lesser extent (other than in the case of visually-impaired children), touch plays a secondary role. The importance of 'proprioceptive channels' is a subject of ongoing debate. Liberman and his colleagues published a classic paper in 1967 in which they claimed that proprioceptive feedback was an essential component of comprehension. But conflicting evidence is provided by instances of anarthric children with well developed comprehension (Bishop, Byers Brown and Robson, 1990). It is most likely that proprioceptive channels act mainly to ensure maintenance of speech, whilst auditory pathways play a very important part in language acquisition. The respective roles of the two modes of input is well illustrated in the case of remedial programmes for people with acquired hearing loss. Segmental aspects of speech can be maintained to some extent through tactile and proprioceptive input, but non-segmental (prosodic) elements pose difficulties and reliance then has to be placed on visual models as in the use of instrumentation such as Visispeech.

Incoming information is held briefly in memory storage before it is perceived. Hebb (1972) emphasises the point that perception is more than a complex sensation. Presumably it is the activity of mediating processes that result from sensory input. Luria (1973) describes it as the encoding and synthesis of incoming information, which is then compared with previous experience. This definition also implies a close association with memory. Integration of ongoing sensory input is a point of extreme vulnerability for the developing child. Instances of shaky motor coordination come to mind as, for example, children's early attempts at hopping, climbing stairs, throwing and catching. Whilst the results are manifest in motor response, the mismatch arises from an as yet incomplete synthesis of visual, tactile and proprioceptive input.

Memory

Stelmach (1982) describes three functions associated with memory: 'encoding', 'storage' and 'retrieval'. Encoding is the stage whereby percepts undergo transformation for storage. This information is then stored over a period of time. At one time, memory was described as a two-part process: short-term and long-term. Current views, however, favour the notion of it being on a continuum. Partly corresponding to short-term memory, though not exclusively so, is episodic or working memory. This has been likened to an internal diary that records day-to-day factual events many of which do not need to be retained. Most auditory memory tasks are designed to test this. Conceptual or semantic memory is the internal dictionary. This, as the name suggests, stores concepts and meaning. Episodic memory is vulnerable to decay, but it can, through strategies of rehearsal and reinforcement, be transferred to the greater permanence of conceptual memory. It is generally agreed that there are four types of code involved in memory storage: 'iconic', 'symbolic', 'verbal' and 'motor'. In relation to language, it will be seen that all these codes have an important role.

In semantic memory the information that is stored, as well as verbal codes, includes that which relates to vision, space and movement. There is no one-to-one correspondence with specific linguistic units, although semantic memory does appear to include the coding of linguistic information (Miller, 1984). Memory plays an intrinsic part in the development of cognition and children have to develop critical selection and means of retention of relevant stimuli from the environment. This development is largely involuntary, but experimental work has shown it to be more effective where the input is meaningful. Language acts as a powerful reinforcer for retention. Children with severe learning difficulties may be taught specific strategies for remembering, but they are limited by their inability to apply these, other than to a particular learned situation. Craig and Tulving (1975) examined processes by which retention of memory might take place. They provided a number of stimulus words and asked the subjects to process each one according to a different dimension. In the case of written words they were required to visualise the physical characteristics of size, length, etc.; another type of processing involved the phonological properties of the word and a third focused on meaning. They found there was a significant relationship between the type of processing and the retention of words. Those that were best retained were associated with meaning. This effect was consistent throughout a series of ten studies. The sensory stimulus itself may not be sufficient to lead to recognition. It is dependent on context, previous experience and expectation.

Retrieval includes the accessing and extrapolation of information from memory. Luria (1973) states that retrieval is active and complex in nature. In recalling information, the individual is required to select, from the storage codes, that which is most appropriate for the task in hand.

Children have to learn strategies to develop a system of retrieval from semantic memory. One such stratagem is the categorisation of incoming information into a superordinate structure so that 'dog, cat, horse, etc.' would be coded under the superordinate 'animal'.

At first these categories will relate mainly to concrete objects, but with maturity, more abstract categories will be learned. In relation to association tasks too, there is evidence of maturational change. Very young children (up to around 7 years) respond to a stimulus word with one from a different syntactic category, e.g. biscuit → eat. As language develops, the response becomes paradigmatic, i.e. it is drawn from the same syntactic category: biscuit–cake–pastry (Brown and Berko, 1960). There is some evidence that language-disordered children have difficulty in making this shift and it is speculated that this may be the result of problems of reorganisation in the semantic domain.

Increasing attention has in recent years been focused on 'forgetting'. Whereas it was formerly thought that memory traces simply faded with the passage of time, it has been shown that interference has a deleterious effect on retention. Stelmach, Kelso and Wallace (1975) carried out a study in which subjects were taught a new movement. During the period of rehearsal immediately following, half the sample was assigned a distracting task (counting). There was poorer retention of the movement in these subjects than in the controls. There is an obvious correspondence here with the difficulties that highly distractible children experience in retaining information.

Response

This entails, first, appropriate selection from memory and, secondly, the planning and programming of whichever type of response best fits the event; this may be motor or verbal. In the selection process, the individual must take into account contextual factors, as, for example, the environment, to ensure efficacy. Information about such efficacy is conveyed through two main processes: 'feedback' and 'feedforward' as described earlier.

There is, however, the possibility of including cognitive strategies within such a model that reduces the criticism of automaticity. In relation to the development of memory, for example, Brown (1975) has shown that conscious cognitive strategies will effect progress. Hubbell (1981) describes human information processing as 'a dynamic multiply determined adaptable system response to both outside stimuli and to its own functions' (p. 39).

Information processing models of word perception, recognition and retrieval

It must be remembered that the relationship between cognition and language is not at all clear cut. In fact, Campbell (1979) prefaces a chapter on this subject by describing it as 'a very dark forest indeed. It is not so much a question of not being able to see the wood for the trees: one cannot even see the trees!' (p. 419).

The acquired language model is shown in Coltheart's (1987) discussion of language processing in adults. This work describes a model that has affinities with work on logogens, which has been developed by Morton (1978) and Marslen-Wilson and Tyler (1980). This is known as the cohort model.

At the input level, there is an auditory word recognition system (there are also comparable visual and picture written systems, but these do not concern us here). This is connected to a semantic–cognitive system that acts as a storage resource. This in turn is connected to a production system. The schematic representation of this model as presented by Coltheart is shown in Figure 4.2.

The word recognition system includes a series of word detectors that can be potentially equally activated. When a spoken stimulus occurs an immediate process of analysis starts. Suppose the stimulus is the word 'play'. As soon as the phoneme /p/ is detected all the words *not* beginning with this will be inactivated; similarly when the next element of the cluster /l/ is recognised, further elimination will take place leaving only those likely candidates that have /pl/ in the initial position. This process of analysis continues until the word is complete or recognised. Obviously in many cases it will not be necessary to go through the entire range of detectors for recognition to take place; in such instances context and experience act as facilitators. Highly predictable utterances such as 'Happy Christmas' will be recognised very early on. The model is extended to included analysis of discourse and, to accommodate this,

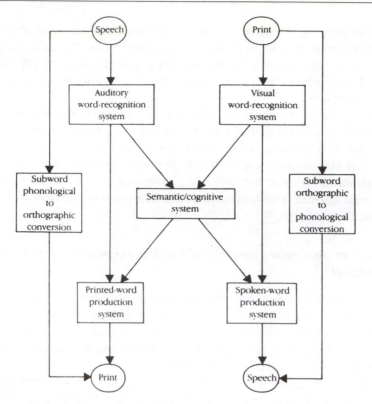

Figure 4.2 An information processing model of language. (From M. Harris and M. Colheart, Eds (1986) *Language Processing in Children and Adults; An Introduction* London, Routledge, Keegan and Paul.)

concurrent syntactic and semantic analysis are thought to take place. There is some doubt about the actual boundaries involved. It is suggested that these may be clausal. It is also not clear whether there is a preliminary phonological analysis followed by a semantic/syntactic sweep. There is, however, a strongly defined interactive component between the levels.

This model favours a top-down processing strategy in that word recognition is influenced by stored previous knowledge and prediction. Bottom-up processing relies on recognition of sound patterns through acoustic cues received. Both methods interact. This can be illustrated by examples of semantic errors. For instance, one student referred consistently in a written paper to a 'raw shark' (Rorscharch) test. She had analysed the acoustic sequence correctly (bottom-up), but because this word had not previously existed in her lexicon, she equated it with two that did, although with minimal semantic accuracy.

An important aspect of information processing in language development was described by McWhinney and Bates (1989) in their 'competition model'. The model takes a purely empirical view of language learning and does not allow for any biological pretuning but, importantly, it gives a good description of 'parallel processing' where different types of information have to be dealt with concurrently. For instance, even to understand or produce a simple utterance a child has to deal with making the right lexical choice, including processing the phonology (pronunciation), the syntactic framework and the pragmatic context. Each language level has several choices that 'compete' with each other, for instance several similes (e.g. words for dogs) in the child's vocabulary. It is suggested that a child's linguistic experience increases the 'activation strength' of certain words for certain contexts so that they are more likely to be chosen. The theory of simultaneous processing of multiple channels is crucial when we come to consider possible points of breakdown in SLI children.

Development of cognitive and language systems

Hubbell (1981) describes the development of cognitive strategies to deal effectively with incoming information as 'a continuum from very automatic activity that may occur almost without awareness ..... to very conscious purposive activity such as that employed in various types of problem solving' (p. 37). These strategies may differ in individuals, for they are learned and may therefore be acquired in different circumstances both within the child and through the environment.

The place of cognition as an underpinning of language has, as one of its chief proponents, the work of Piaget and that of his many followers who view language as an outcome of conceptual developments. The antithesis of this model is that of followers of Skinner who based their ideas around operant conditioning. Thus language learning could be seen as arising out of shaping and reinforcement. Basic units could then be combined to form novel utterances. This type of theory palpably lacks any element of creativity and it cannot stand up as the sole explanation of language learning. However, elements of conditioning are thought to be important in preverbal interactional learning and in theories of 'motherese' (early mother–child interaction), although with a narrow range of influence according to Conti-Ramsden (1990).

Piagetian theorists claim that concepts develop initially independently of language, i.e. they are the outcome of sensorimotor activity. Conceptual knowledge without appropriate linkage with linguistic knowledge is observed in children with predominantly expressive-type language disorders. They may be able to demonstrate that they 'know' an object and that they can differentiate it from other similar objects without being able to signal this knowledge linguistically. Take, for example, a shoe. The child can identify it by form and function. He may be able to differentiate between one shoe and more than one shoe, and from other shoes, all in the absence of knowledge of the appropriate word. The converse of this condition is when a child can use words without having developed corresponding concepts. Obviously, conceptual knowledge at this very basic level will be severely limiting. Examples of this state are seen in some of the case illustrations in Chapter 5.

Piaget views language development as an outcome of cognitive development. Early language and development of representational thought are concurrent but not interdependent (Sinclair de Zwart, 1969). There is thus a firm focus on the sensorimotor period and, in particular, on the motor component of this as a prerequisite for the development of language. In the first stage, language takes the form of illocutionary vocalisations, i.e. they accompany a motor activity. The assumption that the influence of motor activity is all pervasive has been questioned by the evidence of severely physically handicapped children developing normal levels of comprehension (Lenneberg, 1967). Piagetians would argue that a minimal amount of motor activity as, for example, eye movement would constitute sufficient experience. This does, however, appear to stretch the theory to the utmost limits. Language development is therefore regarded as one aspect of the complex of processes taking place, sharing common roots with symbolic play.

At a more complex level of coding, propositional structures are thought to store information about phrases, clauses and sentences, whilst schemata are thought to be concerned with the encoding of discourse size pieces of spoken and written text. Chapter 6 makes reference to Van Kleeck's 1981 review of metalinguistic development within a Piagetian model. For Bruner, the development of language is a much more socially orientated and interactive process. Early vocalisations lead to the building of concepts and as vocabulary increases so the child finds a verbal outlet for their expression (Bruner, 1975).

Cognitive theories of developmental language disorder

Cognitive theories of language disorder propose that the roots of the problem lie with the strategies SLI children use to deal with learning or with their capacity to process information. Some propose specific difficulties with a level of mental representation whilst others suggest there is an overall processing capacity deficit. This has variously been attributed to problems with the memory system itself or memory difficulties due to underlying perceptual abnormalities.

Workers in the Piagetian frame have suggested that language-disordered children have problems mastering certain stages in the development of internal representations, an achievement that is not inborn. Cognitive–linguistic links have been shown to be close, for instance, during the one-word stage of development, where the use of 'gone' appears at a time that the child is mastering the complexities of object permanence (Gopnik, 1988). It has often been suggested that there are particular difficulties with symbolic thought, especially at the level where the symbols, for example gestures, bear little or no relation to the thing that they represent (Kamhi et al., 1988). Others have suggested that deficits in reversibility in concrete operations could explain poor grammatical development especially with word order, although no truly satisfactory Piagetian explanation exists for syntactic development (Flavell, Miller and Miller, 1993) nor is there one for the causal mechanisms of SLI.

The limited information processing capacity model

In this model of SLI it is suggested that these children have a problem in tasks where a strain is placed upon their verbal memory and representational capacities. They fall behind age-matched controls especially where simultaneous processing at multiple levels is involved (Johnston and Smith, 1989). Bishop and Adams (1991) found both comprehension and expressive deficits when SLI children took part in an experiment where they had to hold features of an eight-picture card array in order to differentiate a target and form a message to describe it. Several researchers suggest the underlying factor is actually an overall cognitive limitation that just becomes more apparent due to the demands of verbal processing where the stimulus is transient. Bishop (1992b, 1994) suggests that the speed of normal rates of speech outstrips SLI ability to process incoming information, especially grammatical morphemes. Apparent difficulties in handling non-verbal imagery does seem to be a weakness for SLI children that needs to be explained and once again limited speed of processing in imagery tasks has been suggested and this adds weight to the global deficit argument.

Such theories that propose a global limitation are criticised because it is known SLI children do not have wide ranging cognitive problems. To counteract this it has been pointed out that whilst sensory processing may be poor in early life the problem may resolve and become imperceptible as the child grows. However the early deficit could have a lasting effect.

Other researchers have suggested that the deficit must be confined to verbal processing, for instance in working memory (Kirchner and Klatzky, 1985). More specifically Gathercole and Baddeley (1990, 1993) suggest poor phonological memory. Auditory perceptual or discrimination problems do not give a good account of phonological problems but poorly laid down memory traces due to inefficient processing speeds might yield a stronger model. Gathercole and Baddeley's explanation gives a good account of the trade-off between different levels of language when skills are not automatic: for instance where syntactic complexity is high then phonological errors in speech can increase.

There are some researchers whose work forms a bridge between theories of cognitive and linguistic processing. For instance, using crosslinguistic data, Leonard and fellow workers have put forward the idea that SLI children have difficulty perceiving and processing those elements of syntax that are brief in duration and have little stress, such as certain word endings. The picture is complicated by the fact that they seem to find morphemes that have clear semantic linkage and contextual support much easier to understand. For example, in English the plural 's' appended to nouns is understood more easily than the 's' that represents the third person singular appended to verbs. It is also suggested that languages where morphology is functionally important, e.g. German or Hebrew, lead the children to focus their limited processing capabilities on these areas whereas children learning English, where sentences can often be understood without too much attention being paid to morphology, have more difficulty acquiring this type of linguistic knowledge. See Leonard et al. (1987), Leonard, McGregor and Allen (1992) and Leonard and Dromi (1994).

In conclusion, Bortolini and Leonard (1991) suggest that SLI children simply represent the lower end of the normal language learning continuum and that they simply have a weak set of attributes that do not constitute a different mechanism for language learning. As Judith Johnston states

> I am amongst those who hold that the 'language acquisition device' is nothing more or less than the general information processing capabilities that constitute the mind. From this perspective children can learn the language system by applying their powers of observation, organisation and analysis to the examples of language they hear. (Johnston, 1994, p. 108)

On the other side of the fence stand those theorists who believe in specific linguistic deficits as the underlying substrate of developmental language impairment, and often, concomitantly in the LAD. We will now consider linguistic models of language processing and disorder and see how these fit into the picture.

Linguistic models of language processing

It will be apparent from the foregoing discussion of aspects of human language processing that this is a field that is rife with speculation. Since the mid-1960s there has been a surge of experimental work directed towards an attempt to gain a clearer understanding of its nature. Unfortunately, the published studies have, to some extent because of conflicting findings, only served to emphasise the labyrinthine state that pertains at the present time.

It is, however, generally accepted that any investigation of language behaviour requires a framework in which to place descriptive data. This cannot occur in a vacuum and the case is even stronger when the language under investigation is aberrant. In the absence of such a model, the ultimate aim of achieving some coherence in devising a taxonomy is likely to be jeopardised.

The last section of this chapter offers a very broad model of linguistic programming. Detailed consideration is purposely omitted for the reasons given above. The intention is to provide a model that accommodates the factors, which we know from clinical experience and from empirical work, to be characteristic of developmental language disorders. The model is that devised by Duggirala and Dodd (1991) and reproduced in Dodd (1995). A schematic representation of the model is given in Figure 4.3 and it is one that contends to show particularly well the levels of breakdown that account for subgroups of output disorder. The decision to concentrate on a description of the processes that may underlie language production has been taken because the previous sections have tended to highlight input and storage.

At the conceptual level, the speaker gains an idea of the message that is to be conveyed. It is possible that, at this stage of planning, provision is also included for pragmatic aspects. If the utterance is part of an

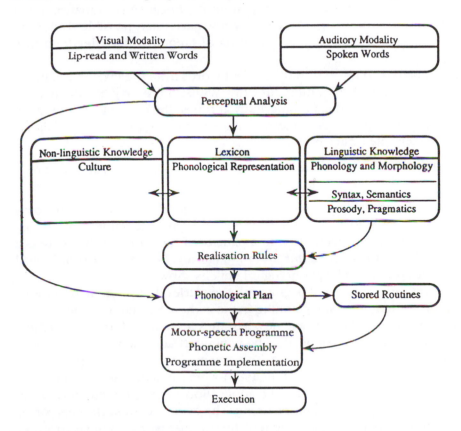

Figure 4.3 Model of the speech-processing chain (based on Duggirala and Dodd, 1991).

ongoing dialogue, feedback will have been forthcoming on listener reaction so that the response or new message will take cognisance of this.

Still at abstract level the next process is the retrieval of codes from the lexicon. These represent the content words in which the message is to be framed. Additionally, a structure for the message is created in terms of their functional semantic relationships inherent in the conceptualisation of the message. One way of expressing these relationships is through terms such as 'agent', 'acted upon (patient)' and 'instrument' (Coltheart, 1987).

John gave	the ball to	Mary
Agent	Instrument	Acted upon

This is not at this stage a syntactic representation for, as yet, planning has not extended to decisions regarding the syntactic form the message will take, e.g. whether passive or active.

Retrieval from semantic memory is vulnerable in that the appropriate conceptual code may be inaccessible or, because of impairment in perceptual processing, storage may not have been possible. Failure at this stage will result in severe forms of language disorder (auditory agnosia).

Impaired ability to retrieve content words from the lexicon will manifest itself as a word-finding difficulty. Whilst there may be adequacy of function words, indeed a superfluity at times, the circumlocutions, hesitations and repetitions can lead to almost unintelligible speech. This is a short example from a boy aged 6;6 years:

The teacher–she had this kind kind of thing –(a pencil) and she do do p...drawed it.

On the other hand some children have a good range of content words but are unable to produce the appropriate syntactic framework, so that speech sounds telegraphic with a paucity of function words. There is a critical link between different language levels as the morphological changes produced by phonological deficits show.

Linguistic processing begins with the retrieval of phonological forms of the content words. A planning frame is then created into which these are inserted. As the message now assumes a syntactic form certain function words and affixes need to be generated and then assimilated into the frame in correct sequence. This brings the processing operation to the propositional level (Garrett, 1980) where it is held in its full phonological form in readiness for the application of the phonetic realisation rules as a prelude to motor planning. The evidence for such rules comes from the consistency that children show across words in the errors they make, as well as the sweeping changes in pronunciation that occur once a rule is suppressed or taught through speech and language therapy. The model also accounts for children's ability to imitate better than they can produce spontaneously as it is possible for perceptual analysis to link to the phonological plan bypassing the child's lexicon and realisation rules. Automatic productions may also possibly be accessed as wholes rather than assembled 'on line'.

Spencer (1986) states that these realisation rules supposedly reflect the child's understanding of their linguistic environment. More recent theories have discounted this belief, for example non-linear phonology (Bernhardt and Gilbert, 1992) and connectionist theories (Stemberger, 1992). Whichever theory is followed they agree that phonological processing rules are useful descriptively but warn against giving these rules any psychological reality for the child.

There is debate as to the size of units of storage for retrieval in the lexicon. Word, syllable and phone have all been cited. The model described above appears to infer storage at word level with the proviso already emphasised here that this is in abstract form. If words were stored in complete phonological form corresponding to surface structure, the phenomenon of a slip of the tongue that occurs frequently in normal speech production, would be difficult to explain.

Dodd (1995) states that we still know very little about the phonological planning of longer utterances. There are differing pressures produced by more complex phonological units as well as those from syntactic and interactional considerations (Kelly and Local, 1989) which produce variation in output. A point at issue is the length of speech that is preplanned at any one time. Halliday (1963) considers this to be the 'tone unit'. This is a stretch of speech lasting over seven or eight syllables with a nuclear stress falling towards the end, usually on a content word. This is signalled by a change in pitch direction. The tone unit acts as an 'envelope' to carry the non-segmental information about the message, i.e. rhythm, intonation and stress. It is likely that these prosodic features are encoded fairly early on in the programme because they both underlie and influence the syntactic and functional form that the utterance will take. It is important to differentiate between prosodic disorder at this level, which is *linguistic* in origin, and that which arises further downstream at the neuromuscular stage, which is *phonetic* in origin. Were this fact more readily recognised, there might be less controversy surrounding the nature of verbal dyspraxia. If the possibility of multifactorial levels of impairment is accepted then the idea of it being both linguistic and motor or either is perfectly compatible with observed data.

The part played by pausing in normal language production casts an interesting light on underlying processing. It is known that spoken language is well interspersed with pauses, hesitations, false starts and repetitions in even the most fluent of speakers. These are not equally spaced, but tend to occur in alternating bursts of non-fluency followed by a fluent stretch. It is thought that during the non-fluent phase there is active preplanning leading to the fluent phase. This type of pausing, of course, differs qualitatively and quantitatively from disorders of fluency arising from neurological conditions. Non-fluency is a well recognised feature of language development and it is interesting to conjecture that this condition, which has in the past been attributed to vocabulary deficit, may in fact reflect the child's development of language processing.

The *motor level* of processing begins with the retrieval of appropriate motor schemata that best fit the message. That all these other language levels interact to influence the final output suggests that there is definitely some form of motor programming that lies outside of the peripheral muscle group (Shaffer, 1992). This too is an abstract process in so far as precise movements are not at this stage prescribed by higher cortical centres. Initiation probably occurs in the precentral motor strip once the linguistic components have been determined, but thereafter the planning relies on influences throughout the central nervous system. Motor schemata, as we have seen in the previous description of neurological function, are concerned with the general pattern of movement necessary to achieve the target. This activity is also under the control of feedback (external and internal) and of feedforward processes so that ongoing adjustments can be made at this covert level.

Impairment in neuromuscular programming may well give rise to dyspraxic-type disorders as well as to those associated with the cerebral palsies. These must be differentiated from lower motor neurone disorders where resulting impairment of the vocal tract prevents adequate production of speech. Such conditions are analogous with structural conditions such as orofacial deformities. At the same time it is important to remember that any of these conditions can co-occur with impairment at other levels in the processing chain.

The motor schemata lead to the planning of the neuromuscular programme that specifies the precise configuration of muscular activity within the entire vocal tract (including respiratory forces) deemed necessary to deliver the message, which at this point becomes overt. External feedback through the sensory channels then occurs and this in turn contributes to revision and/or to the generation of a new message.

Linguistic models of developmental language disorder

In contrast to those who believe there is an overall cognitive deficit of some sort are those authorities who propose that there are innate mechanisms that deal exclusively with language acquisition (the LAD, as proposed by Chomsky, 1986) and can be specifically affected in SLI. Several researchers have proposed that the deficit is 'syntactic' in nature, rather than the children having any difficulty dealing with semantic information *per se*. It has been suggested that pragmatic inference and conceptual knowledge form part of a central, non-modular language system whilst syntax, inflectional morphology and phonology are modular in nature (Sperber and Wilson, 1987; Smith and Tsimpli, 1995). For instance, Clahsen's (1989) theory of 'feature blindness' poses that morphology is an independent feature of grammar, specifically affected in SLI. Gopnik and Crago (1991) have looked at the genetic basis of language disorders through familial studies and shown a deficit in abstract syntactic learning. Van der Lely (1990) investigated SLI children's problems with assigning thematic roles (agent, location etc.) when there was only the grammatical content to help them and no contextual cues. She found a significant deficit in dealing with this type of task where linking rules between grammatical subject/object and their semantic roles in terms of agent/person acted upon, needed to be established. Semantic consequences also arise from this difficulty as word meaning cannot be deduced from the grammatical context in the usual way. Van der Lely has gone further in support of modularity, showing that grammatical SLI children have qualitatively different performance in different domains of language (Van der Lely, 1996).

However, the cross-linguistic studies such as those of Leonard and others (see earlier) tend to favour a more widespread deficit. Innate knowledge parameters for learning grammar have to be very general as it is known that any child can learn any language he or she is exposed to at a young age. Bishop (1992b) concludes that there is not sufficient evidence of specific language components being affected, which could not be explained by a broader cognitive hypothesis. The matter is still open to debate.

In accounting for phonological disorders the universality of processes has again been used to suggest that innate mechanisms are in place. One explanation is that children with phonological disorders have difficulty making sense of and extracting, from their mental lexicon, the rules and constraints that govern the phonology of their language environment. Grundy (1995a) and Gardner (1994) indeed suggest that phonologically-disordered children may pick out totally different features of the phonetic signal as salient for production. Thus tasks that test children's knowledge of 'legal' phonological combinations, phonological awareness and segmentation skills (rhyming and alliteration), show patterns of impairment. Researchers (such as Williams and Chiat, 1993) have studied both individual and groups of children to describe the deficits underlying phonology disorders. Dodd (1995) concludes that there must be multiple patterns of deficits underlying various subgroups of disorder, even if the resulting speech disorder can seem very similar on the surface.

Pragmatic aspects of language processing

This very general description of an information processing approach to language may at times give the impression that it occurs in a semi-vacuum unaffected by outside influences. This is erroneous, for one of the main functions of language is to communicate and, in order for this to be effective, the individual has to be aware of interactive and pragmatic aspects of language. Similarly, he or she has to learn to reflect on the properties of language in order to use it effectively; in other words he must develop a 'metalinguistic' awareness of language. It is now recognised that the interaction between language levels include those at the pragmatic level, not just structural aspects. Prutting and Kirchner (1983) argue persuasively for such a view, in contrast to that which was prevalent in the late 1960s where syntax reigned supreme. The identification of developmental language disorders where pragmatic aspects are central was a natural consequence of these changes.

The position of pragmatic aspects of language in relation to a processing model is problematic but it obviously has a significant role in the generation of an appropriate, intelligible utterance. There are those who regard it as underlying all communicative activity, and as the precursor of all forms of spoken language, for it provides the context in which this can take place; in other words it makes language meaningful. It is perfectly possible to bypass this stage of processing and still produce syntactically and phonologically acceptable utterances, but the word 'utterance' is used advisedly, for there is little communicative intent apparent. (Disorders of pragmatics will be discussed more fully in Chapter 5.)

In contrast to these functionalists there are those who see pragmatics as a separate level of language in parallel with phonology, syntax and semantics. Donahue (1987) argues that they clearly can develop separately. Lund and Duchan (1983) regard a combination of these two views as providing the most fruitful interface between a strictly linguistic and a functional approach. Such aspects have important implications for remediation, and ways in which they can be utilised will be considered in Chapter 7.

In conclusion, the language-disordered population is a multifaceted, heterogeneous one and information processing type models, although having little anatomical reality, give a clear picture of the many levels of language processing that can break down, individually or in tandem. The value of expending so much energy pursuing the ultimate truth, the right model, has been questioned, especially where underlying processing weaknesses can apparently resolve. It is to the question of heterogeneity in developmental language disorders that we now turn.

Chapter 5
The differentiation of clinical subtypes

Summary

This chapter reviews a number of studies that have contributed to the description of developmental language disorders. More recent attempts to delineate subtypes are discussed and commonalities between different models are noted. The last section takes, as a starting point the Rapin and Allen classification, using case studies drawn from the authors' clinical experience as examples.

This chapter will examine some of the clinical subtypes of developmental language disorder as they are presented in the literature and discuss their relationship to the nature of language disorders as described in Chapter 4. Some of the early attempts at differentiation have been indicated in Chapter 1 together with reasons for making such attempts. As was stated in that chapter, the first simple divisions into expressive and receptive language disorders have been found to be unsatisfactory, for such a division cannot comfortably co-exist with the notion of interrelationships amongst linguistic components within a language processing model (Crystal, 1987). Nevertheless, the clinical subtypes that are currently described do tend to follow a receptive–expressive, or input–output, pattern, but the former dichotomy is replaced by a recognition of the effect that one has on the other. Additionally, there is no longer a discrete emphasis on exclusivity of types of language disorder, for as many studies suggest, the boundaries are 'fuzzy'.

The motivations for developing a subtyping system for developmental language disorders, or for other major types of communication impairment, are several. Firstly, and most importantly, it is the transfer and *communication of information* about a child, or a group of children that will be facilitated by such a system. This interchange might occur at a clinical level, with therapists being able to exchange ideas regarding intervention for a particular subtype. It could also be, and one hopes that it should also be, that the subtyping exercise will enhance and promote the further understanding of the nature of developmental language disorders through academic debate and research, which should ultimately lead to more effective assessment and intervention strategies. To date, clinical research and particularly research into the nature of language disorder is 'hampered by the lack of an agreed classificatory system' (Bishop, 1987a).

The requirements of a clinically-useful system of subtyping or classification are, according to Fletcher (1992), that:

1. a number of 'clinically valid subgroups' should emerge;
2. the system should be 'psychometrically adequate'– that is, groups should emerge that correspond to typical profiles of results from standardised tests; and
3. it should be possible to draw up a characteristic linguistic profile for each subtype.

These sound guidelines will serve as a test for adequacy of the schemes described below. In addition it would seem that, for the language clinician, a further criterion would be that the scheme should make *clinical common sense*, and that the individual patterns identified should be recognisable from clinical experience. A daunting task, therefore, for any researcher/clinician, and made even more so by the heterogeneity of the language-impaired population.

Subtyping in acquired language disorders

In the field of acquired aphasia, or the breakdown of language in adults, the differentiation of clinical subtypes has been very helpful to the propagation of clinical techniques. They have generated clear methodologies by which patients can be diagnosed, treated and their progress be appraised. They have contributed to the exchange of information both between disciplines and between international professional bodies because they have provided a framework in which exchanges can take place. Their limitations arise from too strict an adherence to the model so that there is sometimes a tendency to fit all patterns into the framework. Caramazza and Zurif (1978) explore this aspect and conclude that there is no simple or direct relationship between developmental and acquired disorders. However, even though the models generating the subtypes and methodologies may be superseded, the stimulus towards experiment and thought given by the clear differentiation of subtypes has undoubtedly advanced remedial procedures.

We are not yet at the point in the developmental field where a working dialogue can easily be created among professionals because of the subtype structure. It seems that language in dissolution lends itself more easily to analysis than does language in development. Also we can still obtain clearer information from the damaged brain than from the developing one when subjected to neurological investigation. With the increasing sophistication of imaging techniques and growing evidence from cerebral blood flow studies there is the likelihood that increased knowledge will accrue. Geschwind has pointed out (Geschwind and Levitsky, 1968) that 'brains which show no pathology in the usual sense of the term may yet deviate from the normal'. We know that when language users suffer cerebral damage, their language tends to break down in certain ways. We cannot be so sure of the manner in which language is actually acquired. It has yet to be convincingly demonstrated that language-disordered children process language in a different manner from normal children and that the differences in processing are associated with particular types of language disorder. Neither is there overwhelming evidence to suggest that specific impairments in processing lead to specific subtypes of language disorders. However, these are hypotheses we must pursue as we try to make sense of what we find in our clinical population. If we combine these hypotheses and enlarge them to include language processing that is inefficient, rather than aberrant, we can keep some flexibility whilst continuing to search for clarity.

Undoubtedly there are parallels between acquired and developmental language pathology; verbal auditory agnosia, for example, bears some similarity to Wernicke's aphasia. But impairment of development and breakdown of function need to be seen against very different backgrounds. In the case of an adult with an acquired disorder, the breakdown is likely to occur in the context of a previously normal functioning linguistic system so that remnants of this will still be evident in varying degrees. Where language impairment is developmental there is no such background of experience. Different too will be the progress of the condition. Natural processes of maturation will exert influence on developing language, however impaired, so that the pattern of deficit may then change. The adult, on the other hand, may through disease be subject to what Critchley has so eloquently termed 'the drift and dissolution of language'.

The changing profiles of language impairments

When considering clinical subtypes we need therefore to take into consideration the age at which they emerge and their constancy over time. Language delay may herald difficulties with linguistic and behavioural features that only become apparent later. Children who show persistent delay in both comprehension and expression have a poorer prognosis than those in whom difficulties are centred in one aspect or the other (Silva and Ferguson, 1980). This is probably because of the strong association between broad language delay and severe learning difficulties. Bishop and Edmundson (1987a) found that isolated linguistic impairments in young children carried a better prognosis than did more pervasive ones. Haynes and Naidoo (1991), in a longitudinal study of a large cohort of language-disordered children, reported that children whose linguistic difficulties were relatively restricted in range were the individuals who tended to have a better language outcome, thus concurring with Bishop and Edmundson.

Stark, Mellits and Tallal (1983) suggest that some language-delayed children may with maturity show gains in the individual subskills that underpin language as well as in their ability to compensate for specific deficiencies. This view is in accord with their hypothesis that for children with SLI there may be a dissociation between receptive and expressive language. Children who present with a delay in expressive language may master some aspects of language form and then settle into a recalcitrant pattern of phonological disability. Thus over time, *language profiles change* as some functions, e.g. phonology, may remain affected whilst others to which they are related (e.g. syntax) change. The more areas of function that are involved the greater the impairment and the poorer the prognosis. The pattern of disorder will change with development, leaving only the most vulnerable elements still at risk. It follows that if many language functions are initially impaired, then even a shift over time will leave some areas of difficulty. Miller (1991a) describes the *linguistic 'asynchronies'* observable in developmental language impairment and the changes in these asynchronies that take place over time as a result of factors in the child's environment such as intervention and maturation. These fluid, constantly changing portraits of performance impede agreement about a typology of developmental language impairment.

There appears to be a consensus of opinion among investigators that clinical subtypes or patterns of impairment should not be described before around 3 years of age. Aram and Nation (1975) projected their patterns of behaviour from a population of between 3;2 and 6;11 years. Wolfus, Moscovitch and Kinsbourne (1980) used a sample with age range from 4;2 to 7;5 years. Wilson and Risucci (1986) established their clinical classification from a sample with an age range of 3;0–5;1 years. The fact that children with developmental disorders of language do show shifts in pattern over time is emphasised by Rapin and Allen (1983) as they present their own delineation of syndromes of developmental language disorder, based on their findings from data derived from preschool children with severe developmental language disorders.

If subgrouping exercises are to include children as young as 3 years, it is therefore to be expected that there will be a shift in pattern over time. It may be that in the early stages it may not be appropriate to carry out the exercise of classifying. The broad classification offered by Bloom and

Lahey (1978) in which the child's language behaviour is deemed to represent disorders of form, content and use has a good deal to recommend it. This method of looking at language breakdown cuts across the medical models that had previously dominated the field, and was simpler and more immediately effective than the linguistic ones then emerging. Children with different kinds of developmental disabilities could be classified by the methods propagated by Bloom and Lahey and the broad classification could then be amplified by a more detailed description of the child's language. Nevertheless, whilst deserving to stand as a model of useful practice, supported by considerable scholarship, the Bloom–Lahey model did not, in itself, take us far enough in our search to understand all the different ways in which language can fail to develop in young children who are not globally retarded, autistic or hearing-impaired.

In the quest for more detailed typologies, Aram and Nation (1975) undertook one of the first of this new wave of investigations by studying 47 children with developmental language disorders. Their object was to provide some data on an aetiologically heterogeneous sample. Such data could then be used to group children together for classification purposes and to show differential patterns of language. The investigation employed a battery of 14 language tasks taken from standardised tests. Six different patterns of deficit were found from the factor analysis of task scores. They are summarised in the following list:

1. Ability to repeat is better than the ability to comprehend or generate language.
2. There is a non-specific or general formulation–repetition deficit.
3. There is general low performance across all language tasks.
4. There is specific difficulty at the phonological level affecting comprehension, formulation and repetition.
5. Comprehension is impaired in relation to other language skills.
6. There is formulation–repetition deficit with adequate comprehension.

Hearing loss was a disqualification for inclusion in the study, but the authors did not, as later researchers have done, stipulate that overall intelligence must be within normal limits. They did not consider the data then available justified special IQ criteria for inclusion. In 1980 Aram and Nation followed up their original sample, with the primary motivation of investigating the relationship between preschool language disorders and academic difficulties. What they found was that 20% of their sample had WISC scores within the mentally handicapped range and 69% of the remainder were receiving special education of some kind for learning disabilities. The impact of the follow-up data was marred by the inclusion of less than half the original subjects. However, when the outcome for children, classified according to the groups outlined above, was examined it was found that the profiles of children in group 1 had remained relatively static. The next group with pattern 2 deficit were described as 'shifters' with marked changes in strengths and weaknesses. Two-thirds of the pupils in this group were experiencing academic problems. The group 3 children had all continued to show language difficulties and their overall academic level had made them highly represented among those being educated in classes for the mentally handicapped. The inability to substantiate the constancy of the original patterns across time is not surprising considering the attrition in numbers. In their original paper Aram and Nation (1975) state that they have found the classification by differential deficits to be meaningful and clinically useful to themselves, but more widespread application would have to be made before the six patterns could be established. If the patterns proved to be demonstrable only in the original population, it could be that they were associated with the battery of tests used (see Chapter 6). Moreover, as a clinical typology this scheme would fail to meet some of the criteria outlined above, and not surprisingly Aram and Nation's groups are little heard of outside textbooks and academic papers.

Subgrouping developmental language disorders

This section will consider some of the clinical studies that have been published since 1980, in which the authors have attempted to identify specific subgroups of disorder. Areas of commonality amongst the studies will be considered. Recent trends in classification have taken us away from considering whole populations of language-impaired children, and towards more refined analysis-based divisions within an identifiable clinical entity, e.g. expressive language impairment (Miller, 1987, 1991b; Fletcher, 1991). From the standpoint of our own clinical experience through case studies, we will discuss the relationship between some of the subgroups and the language processing model described in Chapter 4.

Rapin and Allen (1983) start from a medical viewpoint by heading their chapter 'Nosological conditions'. Nosology is a medical term that refers to the process of delineating a disease entity. Their data are, however, derived from a number of different sources: clinical data from the charts of approximately 100 children referred for neuropaediatric consultation with the chief complaint of delayed or deviant speech; videotape recordings from approximately 20 preschool children obtained over a 3-year period: formal analysis of the language of 20 school-aged children with severe developmental language disorders; and longitudinal studies of children enrolled in a therapeutic nursery, age range 3–5 years, with a variety of disturbances including autism. The authors state that although the Aram and Nation study was limited to standardised tasks, resemblances can be found between their patterns and some of the syndromes derived independently by them from their study of children's performance under naturalistic conditions.

Rapin and Allen (1983) state that their own syndromes should not be regarded as exhaustive. Their main purpose is to indicate that there is no one diagnosis. Their subjects were grouped according to the most salient characteristics of their expressive language, interactive behaviours and apparent comprehension. The syndromes were then defined by determining which language features were impaired, intact or variable within each subgroup. The authors also challenge the view that language disorders can only be postulated in the presence or near-presence of normal intelligence. They emphasise that the IQ is useful for making distinctions and predictions among normal children, but is much less meaningful when applied to handicapped children whose performance across tests is uneven. They believe that an attempt to study language disorder by looking for a 'pure' form, i.e. one that is not contaminated by low IQ means that investigators will not be considering the majority of children seen by clinicians. Language disorders are also to be found in children with other manifestations of brain dysfunction. This supports the position taken by Aram and Nation (1975). However, Rapin and Allen by moving away from standardised tests make it less likely that they will come up with a group of children with overall low functioning such as that found by Aram and Nation (1975) and also by Silva (1980).

The syndromes that Rapin and Allen described in 1983 were modified by them in 1987, and for clarity it is the revised groups that will be listed here. Some of the labels they introduced then are now in widespread use and in a following section the characteristics of certain key groups will be elaborated and some indication given as to how the profiles of impairment have evolved through the research of other authors:

1. Phonologic–syntactic deficit syndrome: severe deficits in syntax and phonology.
2. Lexical–syntactic deficit syndrome: severe deficits in formulation and word retrieval.
3. Semantic–pragmatic deficit syndrome: deficits in the use of language and word meanings.
4. Verbal dyspraxia: severe impairment of phonology and dysfluency.
5. Phonologic programming deficit syndrome: persistent problems of unintelligibility.
6. Verbal auditory agnosia: severe receptive disorder.

Rapin and Allen (1983, 1987) also include reference to the types of developmental language disorder they observed in preschool autistic children. Of course, many studies of language disorder had specifically excluded autistic children (together with hearing loss and cognitive impairment) as being altogether a separate diagnostic entity. But these authors were interested in a clinical linguistic description of language development and disorder across conventional medical diagnostic categories. Their hypothesis in 1987, which they claim to have found support for, was that the 'communication disorders of autistic children are the same as those of dysphasic children, but that the prevalence of some of the syndromes differs in the two groups'. Other authors, e.g. Cantwell, Baker and Rutter (1978), Bishop (1989), Lister Brook and Bowler (1992) have also shown interest in the way these populations meet and diverge.

At the present time no detailed descriptive data from the Rapin and Allen corpus is available in the public domain. This has rather hampered the process of acceptance of certain categories, whereas other categories appear to have clinical validity as witnessed by their rapid acceptance into the clinical terminology of the day (particularly in the UK). However, their papers have served as a considerable impetus to other workers to flesh out the typology by research into specific subgroups, especially with regard to their further description and breakdown. As a clinically useful scheme, it has the same drawbacks as any other. Most language-impaired children would not fit neatly into one description. But this is likely to remain a constant criticism of any typology, and one which Rapin and Allen address by their recognition of the fact that the edges of the subtypes are not sharply delineated, and that as a child develops she/he may change from one syndrome to another. It is apparent that for the latter claim to be substantiated, there would have to be many more finely constructed syndromes than are currently on offer.

Bishop and Rosenbloom (1987) affirm several of the categories offered by Rapin and Allen and by doing so in a large multidisciplinary text have increased the likelihood of the categories being generally accepted. They agree with the subtype phonological–syntactic syndrome and identify it as relating to specific problems with language form. With regard to semantic–pragmatic syndrome, Bishop and Rosenbloom preferred the term 'disorder' to 'syndrome' for this condition because they believe that a loosely associated set of behaviours relating to language use and content is being described. These they regarded as shading into autism at one extreme and normality at the other. Subsequently Bishop provided the major focus for discussion of the characteristics of semantic–pragmatic disorder (Adams and Bishop, 1989; Bishop and Adams, 1989) and the ongoing debate regarding the relationship between autism and language disorder (Bishop, 1989). There is also an interesting territorial development both in the USA and in the UK with regard to disorders of content and function. If semantic–pragmatic disorder is accepted as a language problem, the child will need the care of language therapists; if it is part of an autistic syndrome, there is less likelihood of the speech-language pathologist becoming involved. Professions do therefore have a vested interest in establishing the precise nature of abnormal language behaviour, but this must not be allowed to detract from the interests of the child.

Wilson and Risucci (1986) refer to the Rapin–Allen model as being clinically derived and imply that its acceptance must await more hard data. They also point out that the Aram and Nation study failed to address issues of their internal or external validity (a notion recognised by the authors in their statement that widespread substantiation would be necessary before the patterns could be accepted). Wilson and Risucci are also critical of another study (Wolfus, Moscovitch and Kinsbourne, 1980), which delineated two subgroups of developmental language disorders on the basis of a variety of neuropsychological and linguistic measures. Wolfus, Moscovitch and Kinsbourne attempted to divide their developmentally language-impaired children into subgroups. They considered one group with syntactic and/or semantic deficit with a view to dividing them into those with deficits in syntax production and those with syntax production and comprehension deficits. It was also proposed to consider whether the broad group could be divided in another way, namely into one group that was semantically normal and another that was semantically impaired. Differences in expressive phonology that could be related to different types of language impairment were also to be investigated. A third aim was to determine whether auditory–perceptual deficits would account for language impairment. This was a topic current in the late 1970s and early 1980s largely due to the continuing work of Tallal, which has been cited previously. Locke's (1980) overview of auditory perceptual assessments is discussed in Chapter 6. The perceptual–cognitive–linguistic battery employed by Wolfus, Moscovitch and Kinsbourne did succeed in achieving some differentiations between groups. Sample size was 19 and the children who had a mean age of 5;7 years had been diagnosed by speech pathologists as being language-disordered. The children were all within the normal range on tests of intelligence. In summary, they found no support for an auditory perceptual basis for language impairment. They found two groups represented within their sample:

1. An expressive group characterised by deficits in the production of syntax and phonology.
2. A group of expressive–receptive impairment characterised by deficits in phonological discrimination, digit span and semantic ability as well as showing global syntactic impairment.

The Wilson–Risucci model (1986) was developed to avoid the inadequacies that those authors considered to be associated with studies relying only on clinical inference. The typology they propose stems from an assessment model that demands the incorporation of psychometric and clinical–observational data. Their classification is based on a branching model rather than on a fixed battery. Thus the investigator can be guided to further investigations and probings by the child's pattern of response. This follows the thinking of those who regard classification as hypothesis testing rather than as an allocation to clinically or theoretically constructed groups. Five groups were hypothesised by the authors on the basis of:

- Consensus among five clinical neuropsychologists.
- Language pathologists' reports.
- Comparison with subgroups defined by a cluster analytical approach.
- Comparison among subgroups on variables not used for classification.

Results are discussed with relation to a number of important issues and a helpful chart is generated showing commonalities with the typologies of Aram and Nation, and Rapin and Allen upon which we will draw. Wilson and Risucci (1986) have in train a number of studies relating to stability, remediation, reading prediction and brain behaviour. They also suggest that indications may be confirmed that will show that the same subtypes in addition to others will be found in further clinical populations including cerebral palsy, hydrocephalus, the Gilles de la Tourette syndrome and learning disabilities.

The 1986 paper by Wilson and Risucci arises from earlier studies (Wilson 1979, 1981) that are not easily available in the UK and this may explain why the work is rarely cited by British speech and language therapists. The constructs used within their tests are, however, familiar as are most of the language and cognitive tests through which they are demonstrated. The constructs are auditory perception, discrimination and cognition (related to levels of auditory semantic comprehension), auditory memory and retrieval, and visual discrimination, visual spatial, visual cognition and visual memory. These constructs as identified in particular combinations give each case its individual profile. The database is very different from that used in other studies cited and the authors point out that it is differences of databases that limit the extent to which commonalities may be inferred.

Wilson and Risucci arrive at these neuropsychological constructs through an assessment procedure in which they employ a number of subtests taken from:

1. Illinois Test of Psycholinguistic Abilities (Kirk, McCarthy and Kirk, 1968).
2. Goldman–Fristoe–Woodcock Test of Auditory Discrimination (Goldman, Fristoe and Woodcock, 1972).
3. Wechsler Preschool and Primary Scales of Intelligence (Wechsler, 1967).

4. McCarthy Scales of Children's Abilities (McCarthy, 1974).
5. Hiskey–Nebraska Test of Learning Aptitude (Hiskey, 1966).
6. Pictorial Test of Intelligence (French, 1964).

Further development of typologies

Since Rapin and Allen's (1987) paper, there have been some attempts to carry on the process of subtyping. However, these have been constrained, necessarily, by the immense size of such an exercise and the resources that are required to support research involving a very large cohort, and consequently have mainly been the byproduct of a specific research project.

Haynes and Naidoo (1991), for the purposes of a longitudinal and informative study of a group of children at a special school in the UK for children with speech and language impairments, subdivided their population into several types. These appear to have clinical validity, at least for this rather special population, and are based on psychometric information as well as anecdotal information from teachers/therapists. In doing this, Haynes and Naidoo derived a system of grouping that 'most nearly conforms to our intuitions about subgroups of language impairment'. It must be stressed that this is not a 'nosology' in the sense of Rapin and Allen, but a subdivision for the purposes of a follow-up study. It should also be noted that Haynes and Naidoo were describing children already of *school age*. The breakdown is as follows:

Speech:	Severe speech production difficulties Minor comprehension/expression problems
Speech Plus:	Severe speech production difficulties Moderately impaired expressive language May have some comprehension problems
Classic:	Severe expressive language impairment Severe/moderate speech production difficulties Mild/moderate impairments of comprehension
Semantic:	Severe/moderate comprehension impairment Expressive language/and or speech superior to comprehension Semantic deficits
Residual/ Moderate:	Moderate impairments of speech/expressive language Poor written language Improved following long periods of therapy
No Language:	Severe auditory comprehension impairment Little/no speech Communication by sign/lipreading May show some degree of improvement in comprehension over time
Severe:	Very severe impairment in all areas. Able to produce single words only

The most numerous group in Haynes and Naidoo's report is the Classic, followed by Semantic and Speech Plus. There are some obvious points of correspondence with Rapin and Allen's proposed categories and these are indicated in Table 5.1, but not exhaustively. Table 5.1 summarises the correspondence between the terminologies employed by all these authors.

In 1987 Bishop had suggested a way forward in typology might be to attempt to describe language behaviours in detail using linguistic parameters (Bishop, 1987a). Inevitably, expressive language lends itself more readily to this kind of depiction and consequently it is in the field of expressive language disorders that recent research has focused. Thus, Miller (1991b) proposed taking measures of 'productive language performance' (for example MLU, number of different words, total number of words) and using these to map out expressive language profiles over time in individuals, thus providing a means of 'documenting different patterns of language disorders'. In 1987 Miller had put forward a typology of language disorders derived from discussion with language clinicians, whom, he said, knew intuitively what kinds of developmental language disorders existed and that there would be characteristic productive language performances associated with them. Fletcher (1992) in an effort to do just this, reanalysed archived data from a heterogeneous group of language-impaired children, making measurements of clause complexity, phrasal structure, errors and fluency. On this basis four groups were differentiated:

Group 1:   fluent
                few speech errors
                adequate clause/phrase structure

Group 2:   dysfluent
                adequate clause/phrase structure
                few errors

Group 3:   dysfluent
                clause and phrase structure problems
                many errors

Group 4:   relatively fluent
                few errors
                clause/phrase structure problems

It is apparent that such exercises are invaluable in the exploration of expressive language disorders and the search for appropriate therapeutic strategies. The limitation of typology to syntactic behaviours, is a byproduct of the ease with which this form of output can be described, compared with input or pragmatic deficits.

Table 5.1 Commonalities of language disorder subtypes

Rapin and Allen (1987)	Aram and Nation (1975)	Wolfus, Moscovitch and Kinsbourne (1980)	Wilson and Risucci (1986)	Haynes and Naidoo (1991)
Verbal auditory agnosia	Generalised low performance	Comprehension + syntactic production	Global disorder	No language
Semantic–pragmatic disorder	Repetition better than comprehension	Comprehension disorder	Auditory–semantic comprehension disorder	Semantic
Verbal dyspraxia	Syntactic and speech programming disorders	Syntactic production difficulty	–	Speech/Speech Plus
Phonological–syntactic deficit	Non-specific formulation repetition deficit	Syntactic production difficulty	Auditory–semantic comprehension + visual short-term memory deficit	Classic
Lexical–syntactic deficit	–	Syntactic production difficulty	Expressive disorder	–

Categories and controversies

Verbal auditory agnosia

Because the block is in the input processing, these children have no comprehension of speech. Whilst they can be distinguished from autistic children by other than language behaviour, e.g. good eye contact, they may develop sufficiently severe secondary symptoms to make the differential diagnosis difficult. This is the one group that appears to have been constantly cited throughout the history of language disorder classification. It is virtually identical to that described by Worster-Drought and Allen in 1930, and subsequently elaborated in a series of publications, and also by Eisenson in 1986. The basis for the condition is stated by Rapin and Allen to be temporal lobe pathology.

This condition has had a degree of consistency of description throughout the literature. It represents an extreme in severity of disorder and in very severe cases prognosis for development of spoken language is poor. Very severe cases are comparatively rare. The term 'verbal auditory agnosia' is essentially a description of the most important symptom and not the condition itself. Eisenson (1985) termed the condition 'developmental aphasia', and it is to this type of severe disorder that the term aphasia in children is best limited. Other reports of children with verbal auditory agnosia have described it in a condition first identified in the 1950s as the Landau–Kleffner syndrome (or acquired aphasia with epilepsy). It may appear out of place to describe an acquired condition in a book about developmental disorders, but in fact, if the condition appears early in childhood, then it is the *development* of language that will be severely affected. The literature available about this group of children therefore suggests that there are two major subgroups of verbal auditory agnosia: one is the Landau–Kleffner type, and the other a non-acquired form, where the deficit is present (as far as can be established) from birth. It is feasible that the latter type might also be acquired via pathological processes in utero or perinatally rather than genetically constituted.

The Landau–Kleffner syndrome has received considerable attention from both the medical profession and researchers. The key characteristic of this condition is the onset associated with epileptic episodes, which may or may not persist. At the same time there is a loss of language, both receptive and expressive. Some children recover some language, whilst in others there is a persisting verbal auditory agnosia and poor progress with output. The prognosis is considered to be more favourable the older the child at onset (Bishop, 1985). A comprehensive review of current issues in this condition is provided by Lees (1993) and a case study of onset at 3;6 by Vance (1991). Further research about verbal auditory agnosia in all its manifestations is needed, but held back by the rarity of the condition.

Whatever the subgroup or aetiology, superficially children with verbal auditory agnosia may appear to be deaf and indeed this misdiagnosis has sometimes been made. This is understandable for characteristically they show little response to auditory stimuli whether linguistic or environmental. The diagnosis is particularly difficult in the 'non-acquired' form. Extensive and in depth assessment of hearing including brain-stem evoked response audiometry tends to show that there is a response to pure tone so that, peripherally, the acoustic signal is received. It would seem that the impairment lies further upstream in the central nervous system, possibly in the association auditory cortex, which as we have seen is concerned with the refinement, recognition and synthesis of incoming signals. Interestingly, despite very thorough early audiological investigation, some of the children have later been found to have varying degrees of sensorineural deafness. How this comes about is a matter of speculation. It has been suggested that as a sort of defence mechanism against the babble of meaningless noise, morphological changes take place within the auditory pathway.

The main difficulty therefore is one of decoding spoken language and as a consequence encoding is also severely affected. Referring to the linguistic model of language processing, there is no possibility of extrapolation and matching from the lexical store for there has been no opportunity to acquire such a store. In other words there is nothing on which language rules can operate.

Behaviourally, particularly in the early stages, the children appear to be emotionally stable and they relate well to other children. Eisenson (1986) endorses this view. It appears as though the complete cut-off of meaningful sound cocoons them and acts as a sort of protective cover against the frustration experienced by children with predominantly production difficulties who are more aware of their limitations. The ability to form good relationships is one of the important aspects that differentiates them from autistic children.

It is obviously very difficult to determine levels of intelligence. Eisenson (1985) maintains that in this condition, which he calls developmental aphasia and equates with verbal auditory agnosia and congenital auditory imperception, intelligence is adequate when measured on non-verbal scales. Our own experience based on a limited number of cases would endorse this view and we see it as representing one of the differential features between mental handicap and auditory agnosia. Some children show good ability for symbolic play without, of course, any verbal interaction. They show a capacity for sustained attention in such activities. These points are best illustrated by reference to the case of a boy aged 4;9 years when first seen at a children's assessment centre.

Y was the second child of Polish parents. The father was an agricultural worker in a very rural part of the British Isles. Birth history was normal as was subsequent motor development. He was described, however, as a very quiet baby who did not babble very much. Hearing was assessed and he was admitted to the Centre wearing two hearing aids. Subsequent testing in a neuro–audio-logical department elicited normal response to pure tones, so the hearing aids were removed.

He presented as an attractive flaxen-haired little boy who if anything was disinhibited in his response to strangers in that he ran to them arms outstretched with a welcoming smile.

He was seen by a clinical psychologist and the Leiter International Performance Scale (Arthur, 1952) was administered. This is a measure that is designed for non-verbal children. On this he performed at low normal level as he also did on the Merrill Palmer tests.

Perceptual testing revealed a gross inability to cross-modally code information. For example, when shown three pictures, a bell, a drum and a shaker he could match the objects to the correct picture in the presence of the object as it was rung, banged or shaken. When the same noise was made behind a screen he was completely unable to identify it with the picture. As well as failure on auditory–visual input there was a similar response on haptic to visual perception. That is to say he could not match shape to pictures or to models by feel. This was particularly unfortunate as it offered little prospect of his acquiring a sign language.

He had no recognisable expressive language, but during play he would emit a continuous noise produced by vibration of his lips. This must have afforded some tactile–kinaesthetic pleasure. The warbling noise varied in length and intonation: sometimes long and high pitched and sometimes staccato. It did not appear to have any communicative function, but was an accompaniment to activity. Attempts at improving awareness of sound met with disappointing results. Obviously this case represents one of the most severe manifestations of the syndrome. He was eventually transferred to a special school for children with severe learning disability. This was in the days before widespread use of computer-based learning. It would have been interesting to have seen how much progress might have been made on a purely visual programme.

A minimally less daunting case was J who was 4;3 years when first seen:

He was able to respond to environmental sound, but not to spoken language. Cognitive ability was assessed at low average. Hearing was normal. J had no recognisable spoken language and unlike Y he was not outgoing, though his severe disability was not reflected in behavioural problems. Cross-modal testing revealed a similar inability to relate visual to auditory input but he was able to link haptic and visual stimuli.

Initially therapy concentrated on linking sound and vision through mirror work whereby the psychologist or therapist modelled noises and he attempted to copy them. This met with little success and it was obvious that the method was the cause of increasing frustration. It was therefore decided to teach a very simple sign language based on the shapes that he was able to recognise. The work started initially with three shapes: a circle representing mother, a square representing himself and a triangle that signified food, the last chosen for reasons of high motivation. At a very basic level he was therefore taught to 'ask mother for food'; successful sequencing of these symbols brought a reward. The basic language was gradually elaborated, but unfortunately the eventual outcome is not known. It is possible that he would have been a good candidate for one of the systems of alternative communication that were then in their infancy.

Such cases to some extent resemble Morley's 1973 study of Sally, the main differences being that Sally had a confirmed hearing loss from the outset and that she was eventually able to acquire spoken language although this was limited by comprehension difficulties. There is also a similarity in the changed states of her peripheral hearing. This deteriorated over the years. Most of the studies rely on single cases because of their rarity. Ward and Kellett (1982) reported on eight children who suffered auditory imperception. There was some evidence of hearing loss and/or abnormal response to sound throughout the group. These authors also identified a further group as having comprehension deficits without auditory imperception. On language measures (Reynell Developmental Language Scales, RDLS; Reynell, 1977) both groups showed similarity, and following intervention both showed similar gains –15 months and 13 months respectively. The differentiating feature between the two groups lay in their response to sound. This suggests two possibilities, the first that the group designated auditory agnosia may be further divided into a subcategory in which the comprehension problems stem from other causes. The second possibility is that the 'comprehension only' group represents an interface between auditory imperception and syntactic–phonological deficit. This study does not provide data on other aspects of perception but it may well be that integrative aspects were impaired in the comprehension group. In relation to age, of the 16 children in the two groups, eight were under 3 years when first assessed and one was under 4 years. Reference has been made to the difficulties faced in subtyping children before the age of 3 years and in this study follow-up data would be of considerable interest.

Semantic–pragmatic language disorder

When Rapin and Allen announced their 'syndromes' in 1983, this was the first mention of the currently controversial category of 'semantic–pragmatic language disorder', as it later came to be known. Their account is as follows:

> These children have fluent expressive language, but it is not really communicative. (This may be true of the early years, but later the picture changes.) Comprehension of discourse is impaired though short units may be understood. Echolalia may be present. The syndrome has been observed in children with hydrocephalus, but may also be present in children without other evidence of brain dysfunction. These children's use of social or stereotyped utterances lacking in content or originality has led to the term 'cocktail party syndrome' (Tew, 1979). In hydrocephalic children, the semantic–pragmatic syndrome may accompany cognitive impairment. The site of major pathology is the subcortical white matter affecting intrahemispherical pathways.

Although in the 1987 classification Rapin and Allen place this at the end, probably in relation to their subsequent discussion of autism, if, as has been indicated, pragmatic aspects of language need to be considered at a very early stage because they are closely interwoven with semantic features, it seems appropriate to consider this subtype as following on from receptive disorders. In the present decade, semantic–pragmatic (SP) language disorder has increasingly been recognised without the presence of a specific pathology such as hydrocephalus and the term is now seemingly used to describe a wide variety of children's pragmatic deficits. The term 'SP language disorder' has thus evolved far from the original description.

Children with this type of disorder have been noted and described for a number of years under various labels. Reynell (1969) refers to them as 'non-creative speakers'. In other references they have been labelled as having elaborated echoic behaviour and some workers have identified the condition as being synonymous with the language deficits of autism (see correspondence in the *College of Speech Therapists Bulletin*, February and May 1988) and Lister Brook and Bowler (1992). Rapin and Allen, however, regarded it as a subtype which may be a feature of autistic language, but that is not tantamount to stating that all children with this type of deficit are autistic.

Controversy has surrounded the characterisation of this group since 1987, on three major fronts:

1. the degree of overlap of features with high-level autism;
2. the variation in presentation of symptoms;
3. the common characteristics of pragmatic impairment that are shared with other language-disordered groups.

Rapin and Allen described this group as presenting with the following features: verbose, with sophisticated vocabularies, but with examples of bizarre, tangential language. Expression is often in advance of comprehension, the children may be conceptually rigid and are generally poor at making inferences. A further characteristic is one of mild social abnormalities (this reinforces controversy 1 above). Rapin and Allen were describing a preschool group. From clinical experience it is apparent that these children may show behavioural and language symptoms that might make differential diagnosis difficult. For example a 3-year-old might present with echolalia (including delayed echoing, which appears most bizarre when stripped from its context), poor comprehension, listening and attention and some repetitive non-verbal behaviour as well as a lack of imaginative play. In later years that same child may appear unrecognisable as a verbose, chatty, but slightly odd child with problems of high-level comprehension and normal social ability. This is one condition, therefore, where to fully comprehend the language processes that are affected it is necessary to bear in mind the importance of the age of the child and the amount of progress that has been made over time.

Further research with these children has featured older children where the condition is more clearly defined. Adams and Bishop (1989) and Bishop and Adams (1989) studied a group of SP children in comparison with 'other language-disordered children' and normally developing children. The objective of the research was to find optimal methods of assessment for the first group. Standardised methods of testing language do not, in general, encompass measures of pragmatics or semantics, and moreover, the noted bizarre features tend to disappear under formal testing conditions. Bishop and Adams, therefore, turned to a non-standardised procedure, conversation analysis, in an attempt to describe the linguistic features of the SP group. They found that this group could be distinguished from other SLI children by certain pragmatic characteristics, but that it was notable that these SP children presented with a wide range of syntactic, semantic and pragmatic impairments. The characteristics that made the SP group stand out were, a high rate of inappropriacy in their conversational speech, and a relatively poor ability to gauge the amount of information to provide for the listener. Bishop and Adams conclude that 'they show persistent conversational features that are not normal at any age, at least above 4 years old'. Here then is some empirical support for Rapin and Allen's description. Other features described in 1987 were not borne out. For instance Bishop and Adams found no evidence for verbosity in the 14 SP children as a group, but reported that certain individuals in the group had a verbose style, often accompanied by poor turn-taking skills. As a group SP children had a high rate of initiation, but not a significantly greater number of utterances per turn than other SLI children (Adams and Bishop, 1989; Bishop and Adams, 1989).

Clinical anecdotal descriptions of SP disorder have also been forth-coming. Smedley (1990), from a pedagogic viewpoint, describes the most frequently observed language behaviours of these children as being: word-finding difficulty, problems with sentence formulation, with the language of time and causality, and of conceptual rigidity. The first two characteristics are seen in other subgroups of language-impaired children, and are not distinguishing features, but nevertheless from a remedial stance they are of significance.

The following case examples will serve to illustrate the descriptions from the literature.

F was aged 4;6 when first seen. He was the youngest of three boys, the other two having no history of language disorder. Birth was normal at full term, but there was a delay of circa 5 minutes in establishing respiration. Information supplied by the referring speech and language therapist reported no feeding or swallowing difficulties. Onset of speech was delayed and he was reported not to use sounds with meaning until after 2 years. He produced odd words just before his third birthday. By the age 4;0 years there was a sudden spurt and within a few months he was said to be using fully intelligible complex sentences, including question forms. There were some word reversals when seen at the assessment centre, language was fluent and well developed in structure, but content was inappropriate. There were a few immature phonolog-ical features. Dyadic communication was largely echoic, but normal language was heard when he was re-enacting fantasies. Examples of inappropriate content taken from recordings made at the time include:

Mother: We saw Lorraine
F: Yes it's raining (it wasn't) Put up the Barricades
M: What happened last night?
F: Happened last night
M: You fell out of bed didn't you?
F: Yes you fell out of bed.

Receptive language was limited. He had difficulty in following complex commands. He could not match pictures, objects or animals. Concepts of colour, size or number were not developed.

The psychologist reported that on the Griffiths Developmental Scale he scored at the 5;0 year level on performance tasks. In the hearing and speech section he was down to 3;0 and 4;0 and managed only a few items. He was estimated to be a boy of normal intelligence on tests that did not require complex comprehension. Beyond simple questions his language broke down and became echoic.

It appears that F has a poorly developed conceptual system. He perceives language and is able to retain a certain amount of linguistic information. What one hears seems to be an elaborated echoic language that has bypassed semantic levels. Obviously pragmatic features are deficient, but one would tend to regard these as the outcome of the main semantic failure.

The second example is taken from the corpus collected by Bishop and Adams for their 1989 research. This interchange took place between one of the researchers (A) and an 8-year-old child (C) at a special school for the language-disabled. They are discussing holidays:

C: but the day when we went to L, on the way, the–the door broke–broked, but it didn't fell down. It fell down it–it was a draught.

A: it was a draught?

C: YEAH (flat intonation) and daddy shut it quickly–but all of a sudden it would- would closed properly.

A: oh dear

C: it would close-close properly

A: mhm?; so what happened?

C: mummy isn't; mummy's isn't; even if it is a three wheeler

A: mhm

C: yeah (flat intonation); we went on holiday

A: so what happened when the door wouldn't close properly?

C: it DID close properly (very emphatic)
I said it did.
AND
and another way to to L
the exhaust was-
the ex
the silen
the exhaust was rusty

A: oh

C: and the silencer dropped OFF

A: so what did your dad do?

C: well he droved it straight to park and then all of a sudden we ate some picnic.

The overall impression one gains from this extract is that conversational demands placed upon a child are very difficult for children with SP language disorder. The interchange is affected by several pragmatic problems. For instance the adult obviously misinterprets what she assumes to be an informative utterance ('it would closed properly') as giving new information: that is that it didn't close properly, and this leads to a minor dispute later. In addition the apparent non-sequential nature of events reported by the child is confusing for the listener. Furthermore, his evident difficulty in mastering syntax and finding the correct semantic and syntactic formulation to convey the ideas he has adds to the listener's problems of interpretation in real time.

It is possible in the future that more detailed analyses will reveal subgroups within this overall heterogeneous category, which merge into one another, perhaps at one extreme being semantically-impaired (including word-finding difficulties) and at the other pragmatically-impaired (merging into the language and characteristic social profile of the able autistic individual). Clearly there is a need for further research until some consensus of opinion can be reached about SP.

Developmental verbal dyspraxia

Children with verbal dyspraxia are characterised by Rapin and Allen as having extremely dysfluent, effortful speech with grossly deviant phonology. Expression is restricted but in the presence of comprehension within normal limits. They may have overt evidence of neurological involvement, e.g. an accompanying oromotor dyspraxia.

In placing this syndrome next in the sequence of processing, we are undoubtedly entering a minefield of controversy. The areas of dispute lie mainly in relation to the following:

• Phonological vs phonetic errors.
• Intrinsic syntactic problems vs those arising as an outcome of articulatory constraints.
• Intrinsic prosodic problems vs those arising as an outcome of articulatory constraints.

Perhaps it may be most fruitful to begin by defining what we construe to be the nature of developmental dyspraxia. We consider it to be an impairment in the selection, planning and programming of linguistic and of motor schemata for production of language.

There is no evidence of peripheral motor impairment and within the limits of current methods of assessment of verbal comprehension there does not appear to be any deficit at this level. The inclusion of 'selection' as one of the features betokens the possibility of an impairment that may have its origins in higher cortical function. Referring back to the processing model based on Garrett (1980), it will be seen that, at a fairly early stage, retrieval of phonological representations of content words takes place. These are fitted into the linguistic frame. This operation is closely followed by the generation of the framework for function words. Evidence from slips of the tongue data in relation to normal speakers demonstrates that mis-selection can occur very early on in the planning programme. Boomer and Laver (1968) differentiate between slips that indicate a semantic mismatch and those where phonological elements are involved. In the former case there is competition between two semantically associated words /I haven't the sleast idea → slightest and least/, and in the latter there is a sequencing error /plincipal frute →principal flute. This last example shows a transposition of second element cluster. Similar types of realisations have been documented in children with developmental disorders, e.g. /I like treacle fot fot toffee/.

Crary (1984) considers that developmental verbal dyspraxia (DVD) is a more linguistically encompassing disorder than the adult counterpart. He specifies DVD as a group of disorders in which predominant features are differentiated on a continuum. This changes from anterior executive to posterior planning function. Along the continuum there are overlaps with predominantly motor aspects of speech, shading into more linguistic planning features. He states, however, that these variations do not have direct correspondence to specific anatomical sites. The motor–linguistic model supports a description of verbal dyspraxias being on an interface between the dysarthrias and aphasias (Crary, 1993). It is unlikely that it is a unitary disorder and undoubtedly, in some respects, it is difficult to distinguish from the phonological–syntactic disorder described by Rapin and Allen. It may be a matter of degree, for these authors appear to delineate a very severe form in which the child may be virtually mute. Stackhouse (1992) points out that there may well be many cases of less severity, and that it is essential to look for a pattern of symptoms, rather than to diagnose on severity considerations.

Panagos and Bobkoff (1984) also support the view that the disorder originates in higher linguistic programming; in fact they designate it as a cognitive–linguistic disorder. They reject the idea that it is confined to the phonological level and demonstrate convincingly that because of the interactive nature of encoding, which will be discussed further in Chapter 6, pragmatic, semantic and syntactic aspects are involved. A 'pure motor' theory could not allow for this and therefore a motor–cognitive model is accepted. This accords with the views expressed and with the model discussed in the chapter on the nature of language processing. We consider this view to reflect our own clinical findings. It has been noted, for example, in a pilot study carried out by Edwards (1982) that non-segmental aspects of language are adversely affected. In tasks involving change of stress, which also alter speaker's intention, because English is a stress-timed language, these children are unable to signal change of stress with change of meaning. Stress tends to be equal and even. Syntax suffers under the influence of increased complication of phonological patterns and this most commonly involves the deletion of function words: 'she started on her way home' 'she go home'.

Crary in his study of 25 children was able to delineate a hierarchy of difficulty at phonological level. Dominant errors were syntagmatic in nature i.e. they included omissions (dominating the most severe cases), cluster reductions, voicing errors, metathesis and assimilation. Less severe cases included more paradigmatic errors, i.e. substitution. These were more apparent in phrase repetition than in word repetition. Edwards' 1982 sample manifested all these features, although a preponderance of omissions did not emerge. Metathesis, assimilation and voicing errors were dominant.

It has been pointed out that the phonological errors made by dyspraxic children differ from those associated with maturational delay. In the case of cluster reduction, for example, the delay process pattern in /st-/ clusters would be deletion of the fricative; the dyspraxic child may reduce by omitting the second element of the cluster: /stocking → socking/. Similarly voicing errors may be voiced → voiceless or voiceless → voiced, e.g. paper → bader and duck → tuck. This last example illustrates the *inconsistency* that has been described in a number of studies as a salient feature. Similar errors are frequently apparent in written work and many of these children experience difficulty with reading.

Associated motor errors have been noted. Stackhouse (1992) considers it to be 'debatable whether a diagnosis of developmental verbal dyspraxia can be made in the absence of oral dyspraxia'. The word 'associated' is used advisedly for a direct cause–effect explanation is not tenable. Neurophysiological principles (Netsell, 1986) regard motor programming of movement as being distinct from movement for speech. For this reason, remediation that concentrates on exercise of articulatory organs other than in the context of speech, is not likely to be fruitful.

Eleven out of the 13 children in the Edwards' pilot study had concomitant movement impairment. This tendency has led to such children being described as clumsy (Walton, Ellis and Court, 1962; Gubbay, 1975; Gordon and McKinlay, 1980). Their impairment relates to both gross and fine motor activities–hopping, kicking, throwing, threading, etc. Diadochokinetic movement is also affected, as noted by Yoss and Darley (1974a) who regarded this as one of the 'soft' neurological signs in their sample. In a replication of this study (Williams, Ingham and Rosenthal, 1981) this was the only factor of similarity. Aetiology is unclear but there are indications, in some cases, of damage or disorder in the posterior temporal region.

Aram and Nation's studies confirm many of the features described above. Because of the nature of their assessment protocol, this particular constellation was not revealed in the Wilson and Risucci work and they note that had it not included information from clinical observation, disorders of spoken language would not have been observed.

Phonological–syntactic language disorder

This is stated by the Rapin and Allen (1983), (and later by Bishop and Rosenbloom, 1987), to be the most prevalent of the syndromes. It is seen by the authors as showing features similar to the classic expressive disorders described by Morley (1972). The principle impairments are in the phonological and morphological systems. Disturbances may include severely limited use of function words and inflections of nouns and verbs as well as severe limitations of syntactic relations expressed within a single utterance. The impression the listener gains is one of non-fluency (distinct from that of stuttering), of the type described by Miller (1987). The development of verbal comprehension may be delayed in these children, but may be adequate for simple social interaction. Many of these children have other signs of neurological dysfunction, the most prevalent being oromotor dysfunction. However, the fact that the group includes those whose phonological skills are better in repetition than in spontaneous utterance suggests that the deficit lies in motor programming rather than in motor production. Rapin and Allen (1983) discuss the possible neurological correlates, which could be attributable to prefrontal pathology, which encroaches on the motor cortex or possibly to some cortical connections. Where comprehension is defective, the temporal or temporoparietal areas may be suspect.

Rapin and Allen have subdivided their original classification into phonological–programming deficit syndrome and phonological–syntactic syndrome. The former subgroup seems to be a bridge between verbal dyspraxia and the latter subtype. Differences appear to relate mainly to degree of severity. The phonological–syntactic syndrome also in many ways resembles the features of verbal dyspraxia as described here, but Rapin and Allen differentiate it in noting that it is combined with comprehension deficits although these are not as severe as the production disorder. They draw parallels between this condition and Broca's aphasia citing, as evidence, omission of word endings and function words. Bishop and Rosenbloom (1987) question this comparison with evidence that lesions of Broca's area do not always result in this type of aphasia and conversely it is found where there are no lesions in that area. This argument reflects the qualifications that were made at the beginning of this chapter. Wilson and Risucci (1986) regard the disorder as being closely related to deficits in auditory–semantic comprehension and visual short-term memory; in other words they appear to regard the expressive deficit as being secondary to reception although they classify it as expressive–receptive. Adams (1990) found evidence for syntactic comprehension impairments in children with phonological–syntactic disorder who had scored within normal limits on a comprehension test. A group of dyspraxic children performed on the same task like their normal peers. Chapter 7 on intervention discusses further, through case illustration, the blurred nature of the difference between phonological–syntactic disorder and verbal dyspraxia.

R aged 4;11 when first seen conveyed information in telegraphese. Language consisted mainly of content words, and verb tense was invariably the present. A LARSP analysis (Crystal, Fletcher and Garman, 1976) showed that the majority of syntactic structures lay at stage 3 with a predominance of three element clauses: /my daddy car Nada (Granada), that buses single desker (decker)/.

Auditory memory was extremely limited and on the ITPA digit repetition test he scored at the 3;3 year level. He was unable to carry out triple commands–'go to the window, pick up the pencil and bring it to me'. Recall of the Bus Story was fragmented. Colour naming presented severe difficulties although he could match well. This may have been a word-finding difficulty (see next section). He dealt with this problem of which he was very much aware by labelling all colours as purple.

Phonologically, there was evidence of weak syllable deletion, cluster reduction and variability (stairs → sairs → stairs), and also metathesis (deckers → desker). Affricates were realised as fricatives.

In some ways R's disorder resembled that of Ruth described by Chiat and Hirson (1987). Fletcher's discussion of this paper in the same issue raises some interesting points. He considers that Ruth's reasonably good level of comprehension may have been apparent rather than real and he provides possible instances of deficit. Chiat and Hirson advance a tentative explanation for the syntactic and semantic impairment being the result of phonological constraints, but Fletcher comments that within the data there are indications of alternative explanations for this type of disorder; for example, failure at some other point in the system, lexical access or the production analogue of the syntactic parser. He draws upon his current research as evidence that such possibilities should be considered although he concedes that, because of the fact that there is at the present time a paucity of hard evidence about the nature of language processing, the Chiat and Hirson explanation may well be correct.

Chiat and Hirson's case study approach to expressive language disorder was followed by two other papers using this design. Gopnik (1990) sees grammatical problems as resulting from an impairment of the grammatical 'module'– an inherent mechanism in the brain. Fletcher (1992), like Gopnik, reporting data derived from a single case study, describes a child who, amongst other problems, had difficulty with lexical verbs and their arguments, and devotes some time to considering how the picture of expressive language disorder can be built up from a fairly narrow base. He reflects: 'the fact that three different case studies have turned up what look like three different types of impairment only underlines how heterogeneous the expression of the condition of language impairment can be'.

Lexical–syntactic language disorder

Rapin and Allen describe these children as late speakers, but with ultimately normal phonology. Their main deficit lies in word retrieval to the
extent that their speech appears dysfluent, and there are difficulties in
formulation of connected speech, narratives and discourse. Syntax was
felt to be immature rather than deviant, and there are implications for
later language development, particularly with respect to abstract
language. They are thought to be late in developing speech and are said
to be rather quiet infants. There do, however, appear to be two
subgroups that are seen in development:

1. Those who remain quiet and have a sparsity of language with difficulty in retrieving lexical items.
2. Those who have similar word-finding difficulties, but who use a
   variety of word fillers in an effort to retrieve words.

This second subgroup has a similar or even greater output than normal-
speaking children, but much of the content is empty. German has documented this disorder (German, 1985, 1987; German and Simon, 1991).
Her first study was based on work carried out by Wiig and Semel who
include items for assessment of word-finding difficulty in their CELF -R
inventory (Semel, Wiig and Secord, 1987). These were confrontation
naming experiments in which LI performance was compared with normal
controls and with children with learning disabilities but without word-
finding problems. Semantic classes selected were numbers, letters and
colours. These were presented in both sequential and randomised form.
Significant differences were found between the groups, the learning
disabled/word-finding difficulty group performing particularly poorly on
colour and letter naming. This was most apparent when the items were
presented randomly. They also tended to take a much longer time to
complete the tasks. Strategies employed to retrieve a name included a
recital of colours until the correct one was 'found'. German remarks that it
appeared as if the children were sifting through their semantic colour file.
   The second study reported in 1987 investigated word-finding difficulties in conversational situations. It was in this study that the difference
noted above in relation to subgroups was observed. This confirms anecdotal clinical evidence. Word-finding deficits occurring in isolation are
comparatively rare. They usually appear as part of a constellation of
problems. The extract cited on p. 194 of the boy who circumlocuted
because he was unable to retrieve the name that he knew and wanted, is
an example of this, for word finding was only one of his many other
problems.
   An important criterion is of course the fact that the child actually
knows the word he is seeking so that failure to produce it is clearly

attributable to retrieval. Various forms of circumlocution are evident, e.g. describing by function, giving associated words, either paradigmatic or syntagmatic, use of vague words, filled pauses–'this kind of thing, er um' etc. Use of gesture including facial grimacing, incomplete phrases and self-corrections with false starts. German's subjects were in a somewhat older age group, 7;0–12;0 years, but plainly her findings have useful implications for younger children. Children with word-finding difficulties are said to have good comprehension. Whereas the presenting problem is at word level, there is obviously some accompanying degradation of syntax, especially in formulating fluent and complete sentences in real time. In addition, there may be secondary deficits in some children in the area of pragmatics, especially in connected narrative ability and topic management. This correspondence between word retrieval and pragmatic ability, although hinted at by Rapin and Allen in 1983, is poorly understood (see Westby, (1984) for some possible explanations).

Retrieval from semantic memory is hypothesised as being one possible source of the deficit, but it is likely that conceptual organisation may also be a source of error. The so-called 'storage and retrieval hypotheses' have received considerable attention in the literature (Kail et al., 1984; Nippold, 1992). Case studies of children with word-finding disorders are few, but Chiat and Hunt (1993) report the case of a 6-year-old boy with word-finding problems, with additional phonological and semantic errors. Within a language processing framework they describe his problems as possibly stemming from an 'underspecification at the semantic level', which feeds into and interacts with output phonology problems. Thus we can see that the developmental neuropsychological approach is beginning to be of use in determining where in the processing model the particular source of surface language problem behaviours lie. The interactionist/connectionist model of language processing which Chiat and Hunt employed should be one direction for the future in the study of a further puzzling feature of lexical–syntactic disorder and related conditions. Many authors and clinicians over the years have noted the apparent connection between word-finding disabilities and reading failure (Kamhi and Catts, 1989). Though the nature of the common factor underlying these disabilities remains unclear at present it has been suggested that deficits in phonological memory may underlie both problems of learning new vocabulary (Gathercole and Baddeley, 1989) and learning to read.

Phonological disorder

Gibbon and Grunwell (1992) describe phonological disorder as presenting as 'almost completely unintelligible spontaneous speech resulting primarily from consonantal deviation from adult target

pronunciations', though vowel systems can be affected in certain individuals (Stoel-Gammon and Herrington, 1990). A child might be
deemed to have a phonological disorder if he/she remained unintelligible after the typical age when children are usually intelligible to
strangers (say 4 years). A pure phonological disorder would entail that
comprehension is within normal limits, but it is quite likely that expressive syntax will be affected to some degree, even if only marginally.
However, Rapin and Allen do not consider this as a subtype that exists in
isolation and it is certainly difficult to dissociate it from some degree of
concomitant deficit involving other levels of language.

The results of assessment in the study by Edwards et al. (1984) lend
support to this view. Of 191 children who were assessed on three
measures (EAT, TACL and LARSP) only 7.3% were found to have isolated
phonological/articulation deficits. The greatest number scored low on a
combination of EAT and LARSP (42%) followed by all three tests (30.8%).

Crystal (1987) drawing on clinical data demonstrates the interaction
between segmental and non-segmental phonology and grammatical
complexity. Ingram (1987) hypothesises that there is an inverse relationship between vocabulary and phonological development. It is not within
the scope of this text nor is it within the competence of the authors to
consider in detail the range of different types of phonological disability.
Grunwell (1980a, 1981, 1982) probably offers the most authoritative
account. There is also a group of interesting discussion papers by
Hewlett, Grunwell, Milroy, Harris and Cottam and Hawkins (all
published in the *British Journal of Disorders of Communication*, 1985,
Vol. 20).

Table 5.2 provides a summary of salient characteristics associated
with each of the subtypes described above. The description of subtypes

Table 5.2 Summary of salient deviant features in subtypes of language disorders

	Comprehension	Production			Pragmatic
		Semantic	*Syntactic*	*Phonological*	
Verbal auditory agnosia	− − −	− − −	− − −	− − −	− − −
Semantic–pragmatic	− −	− − −	−	+	− − −
Verbal dyspraxia	+	+	− −	− − −	+
Phonological–syntactic	−	+	− −	− −	+
Lexical–syntactic	+	− −	−	+	+

−, Some impairment; − −, moderate impairment; − − −, severe impairment; +, not markedly
impaired.

of language disorder described here is not definitive. It is also recognised that within each type, there are gradations. Clinicians will recognise certain signs within their clinical population. In order to affirm these hypotheses we now need to consider ways in which children's language may be assessed.

Chapter 6
Assessment of developmental language disorders

HILARY GARDNER

Summary

This chapter begins by discussing the justification for assessment. This is followed by a review of different methods and the limitations and strengths of both formal and naturalistic approaches are considered. There then follows a more detailed account of current practice with regard to investigation including profiling methods. Finally, issues of accountability are addressed.

For the majority of speech and language therapists currently in practice, assessment is a routine step in the process of remediation. Following a preliminary interview, decisions are taken as to which measures are likely to be the most appropriate, either to confirm or negate an initial hypothesis regarding the nature of the individual's language disorder. These days therapists are able to select from a wide range of test instruments and the temptation to run the gamut of these, particularly when no clear picture emerges, is understandable. This has not always been the case. The advent of so many tests has only occurred since the early to mid-1960s. Indeed it is reported that one very eminent practitioner maintained that the only equipment a good therapist needed was a pencil and a piece of paper. For someone with vast experience and finely tuned sensitivity this may have sufficed; for lesser beings such resources seem barely adequate.

The justification for assessment

Why therefore is assessment regarded as such an intrinsic part of the therapeutic process? The main reasons may be categorised thus:

- To provide a description of the strengths and weaknesses of the child's linguistic system.
- To offer a prognosis.
- To attempt an explanation for the disorder–a diagnosis.

- To indicate possible methods of intervention.
- To procure comparative data from which change can be measured.
- For purposes of research.
- Disseminating understandable information to other professionals.

To provide descriptive data

The philosophy of testing has undergone radical change in recent years. Just as at one time examinations seemed to be designed to expose ignorance rather than to reveal knowledge, so language tests appeared to be slanted towards error counts, e.g. the Templin Darley articulation test was based on such a model. Stimulus words contained a range of speech sounds in initial medial and final position and these were scored on a right–wrong count. There was no provision for an appraisal of the 'errors' (the Edinburgh Articulation Test (EAT) was one of the earlier ones to include this component) and consequently indications for treatment had to be arrived at by the therapist, often on an intuitive basis.

From this practice we have moved towards a system of profiling the child's language. This entails taking a more global view so that instead of focusing solely on the prevailing difficulty, the need to consider how this may affect other aspects of communicative ability is recognised. This consideration extends to non-linguistic behaviours too, for as has been described in Chapter 1, a language disability may well have a pervasive effect in the much wider context of the child in relation to the environment. In terms of language levels too, discrete impairment is unlikely. For example, what may at first appear as a primary phonological problem can have implications for syntactic, prosodic and possibly semantic and pragmatic aspects (as in Crystal's 'bucket theory', 1987). What we are mainly concerned with now is to try to determine the nature of the child's linguistic system, through thorough profiling of all language levels.

To offer a prognosis

This presents many difficulties in so far as it is influenced (a) by unforeseen variables arising in the course of therapy and (b) by our present state of knowledge. In Chapter 3 we described some of these problems. Chief among them is to decide whether the presenting disorder constitutes a maturational delay and if so will it resolve spontaneously, or whether the child is set on course for a pattern of deviant language development that may prove intractable unless early and appropriate intervention is available. Bishop and Edmundson (1987b) have begun to address this issue as one of the aims of their longitudinal study. Their subjects were a group of 88 children whose language development was a source of concern. They were assessed on a series of language tests at ages of 3;9 and 5;5 years. Results showed a hierarchy of disorder with the outcome being least favourable for those children with the greatest number of language functions impaired. Isolated impairments such as a pure phonological disorder were more likely to resolve, although it may well be that within this grouping there was considerable variation depending on more subtle patterns of deficit than their assessment could show. Nearly the whole of Bishop and Edmundson's cohort were reassessed at the age of 15 years (Stothard et al., 1996) and the results show that those children at 5;6 years who were rated as having a good outcome have tended to maintain this into the teenage years. Of those who still had language impairment at 5;6 (poor outcome), 70% continue to fall into the poor outcome category at 15 years. Thus, careful assessment has been shown to be capable of revealing patterns of impairment of considerable predictive value.

When making a prognosis, one must take into account constitutional factors within the child as well as those that impinge environmentally. Wedell (1980) stated that the extent to which a child is motivated to use whatever limited abilities they have determines the degree of their success.

The need for an explanation

Possibly in terms of diagnosis this is regarded as being less important than was the case some years ago, although as discussed in Chapter 4, the underlying mechanics of SLI are still being investigated in order to increase our understanding and enhance remediation. The emphasis on explanations or diagnosis undoubtedly has its roots in the medical model from which early studies of speech pathology derived. Lund (1986), comments on 'the traditional way of conceptualising the problem, which has been to view the disorder as a pathological state' (p. 415). Closely linked to diagnosis is the question of aetiology. It is accepted that at present no cause can be ascribed in the case of many developmental disorders. Bishop and Rosenbloom (1987) in a discussion of causation underline this point and go on to speculate that many language disorders may have a multifactorial basis. Robinson (1987) was able to identify possible causative factors in the group of children he studied, but this was a highly selected group receiving special investigation because of the severity of their language disorder. In such circumstances it is therefore more straightforward to deduce causation from the results of assessment. But even so, there is a need for caution. If the types of language disorder associated with the cerebral palsies were taken as an example, it would not be helpful to assume a direct cause–effect relationship just from the physical condition. Other possibilities, both psychological and neurological, need to be taken into account. Therefore the most that may be posited is an association (Edwards, 1984a).

In a slightly different sense, i.e. non-aetiological, explanations are important. The information obtained from the various assessments, cognitive as well as linguistic, is somewhat akin to the clues of a cross-word puzzle. From each one a meaning must be derived and this, in turn, must relate to the sum total of data so that in the end a composite pattern emerges. Our new-found enthusiasm for descriptive statements should not beguile us into thinking that this is sufficient. We also need to try to discover how the child's linguistic system is operating and why it is thus.

To indicate possible methods of intervention

This is a self-evident fact. The idea of embarking upon therapy on an ad hoc basis would nowadays find little favour in good practice. But at the same time the findings of the initial assessments must not be regarded as inviolate. The term 'diagnostic therapy' has been increasingly used in recent years. Essentially this implies a degree of flexibility in determining the course of intervention (Howell and Dean, 1987). It necessitates an awareness of the changing nature of the child's language and of the interactive effect of the environment on this. A previously silent child, now exercising newly acquired verbal skills may impose considerable change on the attitude of those near to him.

As Wirz (1993) states:

> Without detailed information about individuals and their needs any assessment becomes the analysis of data rather than the assessment of the communication of an individual. One of the characteristics of therapists is that they consider these needs and do not become wooed into thinking of clients as data-producing mechanisms.

Another factor that needs to be taken into account is our own changing view of the nature of language disorder for this too will influence our methods during assessment and even during the course of treatment (Gardner, 1995). Damico (1988) offers a descriptive case study in which with a great deal of unjustified self-criticism he recounts his failure to recognise specific aspects of the language disorder of a child referred to him over a decade previously. The child was treated and subsequently discharged after satisfactory progress, and then reappeared 6 years later with severe unresolved deficits that had previously been overlooked. According to the state of knowledge at the time of original referral, Damico's intervention was probably appropriate. We are all subject to a revision of our strategies and techniques in the light of on-going findings from research.

Olswang and Bain (1996), examined current assessment methods in speech and language therapy, contrasting what they termed 'static' assessments (largely testing procedures and linguistic profiling), with 'dynamic' procedures, which are designed to tap the child's readiness to learn and acquire new forms or new structures. Experienced clinicians always incorporate dynamic assessment into their investigation of a child, though they may not recognise it as such. Olswang and Bain's findings that dynamic assessments were far more predictive of language production changes in small children than static assessments, is hardly surprising. But the results serve as a reminder that this part of assessment is of equal importance as diagnostic procedures.

Many assessments in current use have been developed as part of specific treatment programmes, for example, phonological programmes such as Metaphon (Dean et al., 1990), or language programmes such as the Derbyshire Language Scheme (Knowles and Masidlover, 1987). Careful screening assessment must take place prior to these in order that the child is fitted into a suitable treatment programme rather than one that is inappropriate to his or her needs.

To procure comparative data from which change can be measured

It is a prime requirement of good practice that the course of therapy that has been undertaken should be monitored and evaluated. This is important both for anticipatory and retrospective reasons; in anticipation so as to determine the steps that should be taken in the future as a result of evaluation, and retrospectively in order to match the outcome against the content of past therapy. In Chapter 3, we have drawn attention to the special nature of monitoring, particularly with reference to ways in which it exceeds the role of re-evaluation.

An additional reason for this is the fact that a child may be subject to a change of therapist. To ensure continuity it is essential that the incoming therapist should have access to complete information regarding assessment and progress in order to minimise possible adverse effects of change. Issues of accountability, which have been touched upon in Chapter 3, also enter into the need for data that measure progress. This has been a stumbling block for some time as there are problems measuring change when the population under scrutiny is so heterogeneous and, as Howard, Hartley and Muller (1995) point out, the qualitative changes that occur can be statistically insignificant but communicatively very significant for that individual. They advocate a single-case study approach to measurement.

For purposes of research

Knowledge about language disorders derived from research studies is still relatively sparse, especially when compared with scientific work emanating from professions of longer standing such as psychology or medicine. Happily there is a perceptible change now taking place with an increase in publication of valuable research both from within the ranks of speech and language therapists on their own and from those collaborating with other professions and disciplines. There is, however, an obligation to record meticulously our findings, strategies of intervention and outcome. This practice enables other workers to benefit and thus enhance the fruitfulness of their own work. Precepts that have been inculcated during undergraduate days should not be abandoned in practice on the pretext of pressure of work. The time-consuming factor is well recognised but for justification that this time is well spent the reader should refer to Crystal (1982a).

Methods of assessment

The preliminary interview

This is of course an important precursor of the form of assessment that may follow. It is not proposed in this text to enter into detailed discussion of interview techniques and procedures. The assumption is made that advanced students will already be familiar with these and that clinicians will in any case be employing them regularly. Guidance can be found in Hubbell (1981, Chapter 7), Miller (1981), Warner, Byers Brown and McCartney (1984) and Barrows and Pickell (1991). Checklists such as that of Gerard (1986) also provide a useful basis for the interview.

Additional points that it may be useful to bear in mind are: it will not necessarily be the mother who provides biographical information about the child. Quite apart from those cases where the child for one reason or another is not living with the natural parents, changing cultural patterns may mean that the therapist's first line of contact will be with the father or step-parent. It is also very possible that the child may come from a home where English is not the mother language and this could present problems for interviewing. There is considerable variation in pragmatic behaviours between differing cultures and a mismatch between the intention of the speaker and the code of the listener can give rise to misunderstanding. Interpreters are more easily available these days and their use is best served by ensuring an adequate pre-interview briefing in the precise nature of the information required.

It is very likely that referral for speech and language therapy represents one link in a chain of previous referrals. There is therefore a need to establish, in advance if possible, what these other links are and to ascertain what information was obtained then. Because of the nature of language disorders, the therapist is probably functioning as a member of a team and good communication channels are an essential part of good practice.

There is considerable pressure on therapists in busy clinics and schools to make accurate assessment of a child's needs from one or two appointments. However, where treatment is to ensue the interview need not be viewed as a once-and-for-all occasion. Present practice favours active participation of parents in remediation and this should afford ample opportunity in the ongoing situation to obtain further information or to confirm or revise that previously given.

Descriptive language data

The following section deals specifically with assessment of language. It would, however, be wrong to regard this as a discrete entity. Language represents one very important aspect of behaviour that must be seen in relation to cognitive, emotional and social factors. Some aspects of these will have been deduced by the therapist in initial encounters with the child and from observation with the care-giver. Some characteristics of children who have impaired language are described in Chapter 1. There are two broadly defined methods commonly in use whereby detailed information about children's language may be obtained. These fall under the headings of:

1. Formal language testing.
2. Observational procedures (spontaneous language sampling).

Contrary to some expressed beliefs, these two methods are not mutually exclusive. Each method stands in complementary relationship to the other. Each has its limitations and even if taken in conjunction they may not produce a definitive index of a particular pattern of language disorder. But they do serve as valuable pointers to the direction of remediation even though in the light of on-going treatment and growth in depth of knowledge of the child's language system, initial impressions may be modified.

Formal tests

These can be divided into:

1. Norm-referenced tests.
2. Criterion-referenced tests.

During the early and mid-1960s there was a marked increase in the number and type of standardised language tests. For example, two which were in common use are the Illinois Test of Psycholinguistic Abilities (ITPA; Kirk, McCarthy and Kirk, 1968) and the Reynell Developmental Language Scales (RDLS; Reynell, 1977). The format of the latter has proved so popular that it is soon to be revised, taking into account more recent theoretical considerations.

Almost invariably, these are normative referenced tests, that is to say, they compare an individual's performance with that of a number of other children matched for age and given the same tasks. Results of these tests are reported in standard scores and the number of standard deviations from the mean can then be computed. Alternatively the score can be expressed in percentiles. Some tests also include provision for a language age (e.g. RDLS and Test for Auditory Comprehension of Language (TACL); Carrow, 1973). Other tests rely on reported information, the data being obtained usually by questionnaire. The Vineland Maturity Scale (Doll, 1965) is one example. Here the results are compared with age-related norms.

Such tests have value in identifying the existence of a problem as a first-line method following referral. It is possible that the child will already have had some type of screening test prior to this, for example the checklists produced by AFASIC for both health professionals and teachers. Rescorla, Hadicke-Wiley and Escarce (1993) particularly mention the value of parent reports in screening for language disorder. Such procedures determine whether referral to a speech and language therapist is an appropriate course of action. Reference has been made in Chapter 3 to the advantages and limitations of screening methods. It was pointed out that the multi-district study of Edwards et al. (1984) revealed only about 10% of inappropriate referrals. These findings were based on results of two standardised tests that were given at the initial assessment. Scores obtained on the EAT (Anthony et al., 1971) and on the TACL were tabulated against referring agents. A score of at least one standard deviation on either or both of these was taken to indicate a need for further investigation. On this basis, only 10.9% were found not to require further assessment. These 10.9% may have included children whose difficulties were not revealed by the tests, e.g. a disorder confined to syntactic level only, although this is unlikely. It might also be argued that the results showed selection bias in that therapists would hesitate to refer children in whom they did not observe deficits. There is also the possibility that children whose language problems were of a subtle nature were overlooked. Nevertheless, this low figure of 'no problem' does give confidence that, whatever screening methods were in use by referring agents, they were, and still are, reasonably effective.

Formal tests if well designed will offer categorical evidence of deficit, but will be unlikely to elucidate its precise nature. As Lees and Urwin (1991) point out two children can fail an item for very different reasons. For example failure on one of the lengthy instructions in the RDLS does not show whether it was due to auditory memory difficulty, poor vocabulary or conceptual development. However, assessments such as the Test for Reception of Grammar (TROG; Bishop, 1983) overcome this by targeting specific syntactical categories in each item. Other assessments that are weak in providing qualitative information are those such as the

British Picture Vocabulary Scales, which gives a quantitative rather than qualitative picture and the EAT, which gives no idea of the child's system of meaningful contrasts. Reliance on standard scores may also give a false picture of actual progress. This was apparent in the above-mentioned research study and was well exemplified by the case of a boy whose standard score at first assessment on the EAT was 67. Eighteen months later it was actually lower at 62. The qualitative analysis, however, showed a significant move towards more mature realisations. At the first assessment he produced 30 atypical (i.e. deviant and non-attributable to maturational lag) sounds. Eighteen months later this figure was reduced to 11. Similarly in the 'very immature' category, the initial figure of 16 was reduced to 12. 'immature sounds', a less severe category, had however increased from four to 14 and there were now two 'almost mature' realisations. The pattern therefore was one of progression towards an adult system, but none of these changes could be reflected in the total score because this only recognises adult realisations.

A frequently cited fact in favour of standard tests is that of objectivity, but as Muma (1978) observes, objectivity may be at the expense of relevance. However impeccable they may be in terms of validity and reliability, they do impose upon the child an artificial context in which he is required to demonstrate his understanding and/or use of language. Such artificiality applies not only to the content of the test but also to the setting in which it is given and this may have an indirect effect on results (Leonard et al., 1978). Neither is a one-off test likely to produce a true picture of the child's communicative ability. Byers Brown (1985) observed that:

> Screening for communication problems in infants is not a simple matter of counting response, but rather of putting together a number of observations, collecting evidence along a spectrum and not coming to a decision upon one pass/fail criterion. (p. 10)

It has also been shown, through analysis of interactional style, that professionals are not as objective in testing as they may think. They actually respond differently to correct and incorrect responses and give other cues as to the child's performance that are difficult to exclude from the testing situation (Marlaire and Maynard, 1990).

Interaction of linguistic levels

Damico (1988) attributes his failure to recognise the true nature of his patient's language disorder, in part, to the tradition whereby language tests fragment levels into discrete components without recognition of the strong evidence against the autonomy of linguistic levels.

Crystal (1987) writes compellingly of the need to pay attention to the interaction of the different levels as well as to what is taking place at each level. Drawing on reports from a number of studies, he goes on to describe some of the possible interactions that can take place, for example, syntax/semantics/pragmatics; syntax/non-segmental/segmental phonology. Recent work has attempted to delineate subgroups of language reflecting this interaction and these were the basis of discussion in Chapter 5.

Formal tests are unable to demonstrate these aspects; it is only through descriptive methods that they can be effectively charted. Profiles such as Phonological Assessment of Child Speech (PACS; Grunwell, 1985) and the Bristol Language Development Scales (Gutfreund, Harrison and Wells, 1989) make attempts to chart the comparative development of different levels of language.

Tests that rely on developmental milestones have long been shown to have low validity (Weiner and Hoock, 1973). This reliance is based on the fallacy that children develop in a uniform linear fashion acquiring certain skills within given temporal parameters. Similarly, tests that relate to a posited language age are not really very helpful. In terms of design they are weak. One reason for this may be because at the lower age limit there are customarily more items than at upper limits. This of course reflects the more rapid changes that occur during early language development. Therefore a 1-year delay at chronological age 4;0 years may be the result of failure on as many as 12 items, whereas a 1-year delay at age 10;0 years may involve failure on only one or two items (McCauley and Swisher, 1984). Results are also misleading in that language age does not accurately mirror the child's language system. Take, for example, the case of a 5-year-old child who is stated to have a language age equivalence of 3 years. His or her language will not precisely replicate that of a normal 3-year-old. In some respects it will be more advanced by virtue of added life experience; in others it may be more retarded. Strategies that may have developed along the line to cope with the deficit will also have an effect which is not age-related on language.

Strengths of formal tests

So, it might be asked, does a language test have any value? Provided that certain criteria are met it has a place in clinical assessment. First and foremost is the question of selection. Well-designed tests will have an accompanying manual describing in detail the population on which they have been standardised, the purpose for which they are intended and the sensitivity of the different subtests. Cultural differences may well influence performance and so this needs to be borne in mind. For example many American-English tests available in this country have items that do not directly translate into English. Obviously there are also problems for the many ethnic groups in this country using English as a second language, especially in the early years. Familiarity with the contents of the manual is absolutely mandatory if credence is to be placed in quantifiable results. After careful study we should be left with a clear indication of the appropriateness of the instrument for a particular individual.

Secondly, instructions for administration of the test must be followed rigorously. Therapeutic leanings are sometimes at variance with this precept, and knowledge of the child can lead towards securing an enhanced score. Whilst this may be acceptable sometimes when employing naturalistic methods, objectivity is a strict criterion of formal testing. It is also important to remember that the resulting data give information about the child's language as it relates to the model on which the test is based. Another test designed on a different model may yield different results (see, for example, discussion in Bishop, 1986).

Summary

The use of norm-referenced tests will have the following advantages:

- As a first line measure to determine the extent although not necessarily the nature of the problem.
- To give an indication of the direction that subsequent more detailed investigation should take.
- To provide safeguards against variability in replication. This means that a child who has been tested on one occasion should be able to be retested with confidence by another user with the same test.
- To yield interpretable data for use in any estimates of accountability and effectiveness of therapy to other professionals.
- Usually quick and easy to administer.

Norm-referenced tests must nevertheless be regarded as adjuncts to other methods, for it is patterns of behaviour rather than levels of performance that determine how an individual functions linguistically.

Criterion-referenced tests

These differ from norm-referenced assessments in that comparative data are measured within the individual rather than against a hypothesised norm. Their purpose is to chart the changing language patterns of the child relative to certain predetermined tasks or goals (Bloom and Lahey, 1978). They are particularly valuable as reassessment measures during treatment in that they enable the clinician to estimate the stability of a specific linguistic behaviour that has been taught. Miller (1981) uses elicited imitation tasks for this purpose.

Until recently, criterion-referenced tests have not enjoyed the same degree of popularity as norm-referenced tests although there are some published assessment procedures that have a criterion-referenced component, for example the TOWK assessment of semantics (Test of Word Knowledge; Wiig and Secord, 1992).

Formal tests are undoubtedly easier to administer, because specific directions as to procedures are laid down and raw scores can be obtained, converted into standard scores, percentiles or ranked. Criterion-referenced measures on the other hand demand a very solid basis of knowledge of the developing language system on the part of the assessor. In other words, there is a need to be very certain that the targets being set are appropriate. There is also a requirement for ingenuity in designing protocols through which it is possible to determine whether the target is being achieved. As a corollary to this goes the necessity of meticulous record keeping of which language profiles must play a part. If, for example, the aim is to teach comprehension of prepositions, we might begin in a circumscribed manner with two contrasts, in/out–using objects as illustration and to provide context. When comprehension of this was stabilised in a particular situation, we might then move on to pictures and thence to wider contexts, proceeding from concrete to abstract situations.

Reference has been made to the use of relatively formal elicitation methods to establish structures, but there is some evidence that correct responses are not thereby generalised to free speech (Prutting, Gallagher and Mulac, 1975). Any reassessment needs to allow for this possibility. The above description indicates that criterion-referenced tests are very much interwoven into the fabric of therapy. Turton (1983) states that one of the criticisms levelled against them is that, because information is obtained in a naturalistic setting, they have neither reliability nor validity. He disputes this view on the grounds that repeated measures of a single behaviour serve to enhance rather than to diminish reliability, whilst the testing of such behaviour in depth confirms validity. Criterion-referenced testing does not carry with it a connotation of failure, such as is sometimes associated with norm-referenced tests in which the child is required to perform ever increasingly difficult tests until a ceiling of failure is reached (Haynes, 1986).

A paper that goes into considerable detail as to the administration of criterion-referenced tests, using the example of adolescent language needs in a school settings, is that of Wiig (1995). Using 10 probes at one skill she describes four levels of acquisition of a particular skill that can be measured in percentage success. Thus the child passes from a chance level (30%), through 'emergence and frustration' (30–50%) a transitional level (50–80%) to control (80+%). It is possible for children at this age to be involved in self-assessment to some degree as they may have insight into their communication needs.

The need for something other than an 'all or nothing' marking system in formal and informal testing, which gives scope for marking delay, repetition, self-correction, etc has been addressed by Lees and Urwin (1991). This is somewhat simpler than tests such as the PICA (PORCH, 1972), which had 16 levels of response.

Spontaneous language samples

This is the starting point from which the majority of naturalistic assessments are derived. The notion of language sampling has come into prominence in the last decade. Bloom and Lahey (1978), Muma (1978), Miller (1981), Crystal (1982b) Lund and Duchan (1987) and Dollaghan and Campbell (1992) are among those who have developed and refined the methodology. That these naturalistic assessments should also rigorously attend to matters of validity and reliability, much as good formal assessment does, has been emphasised by Adams and Bishop (1989), and McCartney (1993).

Opinions vary as to what constitutes a representative sample both in terms of length and context. There is, however, general agreement that it should include more than one situation. Gallagher (1983), discussing contextual representativeness, considers that this needs to be determined individually for each child and that consequently a decision cannot be made until there has been an extensive pre-assessment to discover habits, interests, etc. This she undertakes by means of a very lengthy questionnaire that is completed by the mother or care-giver.

Wells (1985), for his longitudinal Bristol study which was concerned with normally developing children, probably devised the ultimate method of obtaining as natural a sample as possible. For this, the study children were provided with a specially designed harness fitted with a radio microphone thereby giving them freedom of movement. This was worn during waking hours for a period of 24 hours before the observer visited the home. Thus almost every interchange between mother or care-giver and child was picked up and relayed to a nearby receiver and then transmitted to a tape recorder. These recordings were subsequently transcribed by research linguists. Alas, such sophisticated resources are generally only available for large scale studies.

At a more realistic level a minimum of three situations seems to be generally recommended. Miller (1981) suggests

1. 15 minutes with the mother in free play.
2. 15 minutes with the clinician in free play.
3. 15 minutes with the clinician directing the child with questions and commands.

Presumably the last situation is for the purpose of eliciting specific features and/or estimating the level of verbal comprehension. The notion of providing specific contexts for each child is an attractive one, particularly as it leads easily into intervention. But for research purposes where a large number of subjects may need to be sampled, a more uniform situation is necessary. Most clinicians will have sets of toys that are developed and designed to appeal to both boys and girls. These were used in the study of Edwards et al. (1984); others may use pictures. The Bus Story (Renfrew, 1972b) has proved to be an attractive way of obtaining preliminary information about both comprehension and production of connected speech. This has regained popularity recently.

This type of descriptive assessment has many strengths and some limitations. Chief among the latter is the plea that it is a very time-consuming procedure. McCauley and Swisher (1984) report on a survey in which clinicians were asked about types of assessments used. Whilst many were reported to favour a descriptive approach fewer than one-third actually used this form of analysis. The results of a questionnaire carried out in the UK by Baker (1988) yielded a similar response in relation to various types of language sample analyses: 87.9% of the respondents stated that they would ideally use this method at 6-monthly intervals, but in reality only about 33% of these did so. The time factor was the over-riding reason advanced for this. A significant number stated that they would be helped greatly by computer-assisted analysis. The value of computers may, however, represent a somewhat enhanced view, for as those who are in the habit of analysing language samples well know, it is the transcription that is the most onerous in terms of clinic time and as yet there is no way of avoiding this manual task. This last study suffered from very poor overall return, so the results may not be representative. They are likely to be biased in favour of language sampling, because the therapists attempting this type of assessment would be the most motivated to reply. Much of course depends on where priorities are placed in clinical management. If clinicians bow to pressures of producing figures for statistical returns as a prime requirement, they are in danger of perpetuating a purely technical skills approach to their work. Intervention surely entails more than that and language disorders cannot be treated in a prescriptive manner. That may mean a reduction in overall numbers, but an improvement in the quality of treatment.

Clinicians who adopt a combined approach of formal and descriptive assessment testify to the bettering of subsequent treatment and results. One of the strengths of naturalistic methods is that they allow for a holistic appraisal of the child's communicative behaviour. Reference has already been made to the interrelationship of language levels and to the necessity for assessment measures to take these into account. Muma (1983) maintains that descriptive assessment helps to focus on the individual nature of the child's disability. If an apparent phonological deficit is considered, for example, a sample of spontaneous utterance will provide far more information about a child's language system than will one derived from a set of stimulus words, however representative they may be. Taken in isolation they will be unable to provide information about features such as co-articulation, relationship to morphology or to syntactic complexity. For these reasons we would therefore wish to advocate the combination of both formal and informal methods in any assessment procedure.

Obtaining and interpreting the data

We have described methods by which samples of children's language may be obtained and have discussed the strengths and limitations of different procedures. But this represents only an intermediate stage in the process. A framework in which the data can be placed so as to give positive indications for remediation needs to be formulated. In other words what steps need to be taken in order to make sense from the information obtained and how can the results be translated into goals appropriate to the real-life world of the child?

There are several ways in which an analysis can be undertaken; formal testing, as has been pointed out, is one. Because many of the current tests of this nature have been comprehensively reviewed elsewhere, it is not proposed to consider them in detail here. Readers wishing to study such reviews should turn, for example, to Grunwell (1980b), Muller, Munro and Code (1981), McLaughlin and Gullow (1984) and Beech, Harding and Hilton-Jones (1993).

Profiles

Profiles of children's language have become increasingly popular over recent years. *Chambers Thesaurus* in its 1987 edition gives the following among alternatives for the word 'profile': 'analysis–chart–contour–shape'. In terms of language any of these labels serves well as a description of the data obtained. Profiling has the advantage that it can accommodate many aspects of language: cognitive, linguistic and biological.

Profiles can compare performance on different components of language or target one specific area such as syntax or phonology. A profile such as the Bristol Developmental Language Scales (Gutfreund, Harrison and Wells, 1989) attempts to cover the first three on one form. Others, such as PACS (Grunwell, 1985) cover one specific aspect in detail. The profiles with which British speech and language therapists are likely to be familiar are those devised by Crystal and his colleagues. There are four of these: PRISM, which is concerned with semantics; LARSP, with syntax; PROPH, phonology; and PROP which profiles prosodic features. In the 1982 edition of *Profiling Linguistic Disability*, Crystal (1982b) has an introductory chapter in which he discusses the functions of profiles. They have two principal aims: the first is to identify the (linguistic) level of the child in relation to the level that should be achieved, and the second is to suggest a remedial path. The author emphasises the fact that these profiles do not specify in any way how remedial goals should be devised. In this respect they differ from language programmes that are much more prescriptive in nature and that tend to lack the flexibility necessary if each case is to be treated on an individual basis. Crystal sees the development of profiles as a 'compromise between clinical practice and academic diagnostic research'.

Certainly the flexibility of profiling would appear to be one of its strengths, for it allows for investigation at a series of different levels of detail: what has been termed both molar and molecular analysis. From the first broad transcription, areas of particular difficulty can be pinpointed and these in turn can then be further investigated.

At this stage, profiling systems that are adequate to assess all the processes described in Chapter 4 have not yet been developed. There is, for example no effective way in which the components of verbal comprehension can be profiled and therefore, pending outcome of research in this highly complex field, reliance is still placed upon tests. Therefore a balance has to be sought in using the best kind of assessment for each facet of language, restricting highly detailed profiling and analysis to those areas requiring thorough investigation. Howlin and Kendall (1991), and Stackhouse and Wells (1993) particularly advocate the methodology of broad-based profiles made up from formal and informal assessment procedures.

Components of language disorder

One possible framework within which the components of developmental language disorders can be assessed is shown in Table 6.1. This is based on the psycholinguistic, information processing models that are described in Chapter 4. As Stackhouse and Wells (1993) point out it is necessary to distinguish, not only between input and output processes, but between those that tap into the child's stored linguistic knowledge (i.e. 'internal representations') and those that require the child to deal with sensory, perceptual and kinaesthetic stimuli (both input and output).

Table 6.1 Components of language assessment

Input	Internal representation	Output
Prelinguistic attention and perception	Perception	Pragmatics (as the speaker)
Pragmatics (as the listener)	Episodic memory	Linguistic planning(lexical/ grammatical and phonological)
Linguistic segmentation	Long-term (semantic) storage	Motor planning (articulatory)
Comprehension	Concept formation	

Pragmatics

An awareness of the importance of this aspect of communication has been slow to emerge but now there are formal and informal protocols available to aid assessment. For a detailed account of this area of clinical skill see Smith and Leinonen (1992). One of the first, Prutting (1982, cited in Prutting and Kirchner, 1983) developed a protocol that covers four broad areas of pragmatics. These are:

- The utterance act: this relates to the way in which the act is presented, for example, the degree of fluency, voice quality, body language, etc.
- The prepositional act, which includes the linguistic aspects of the utterance, lexical choice, word order, contrastive stress.
- The illocutionary act, which conveys the speaker's intention.
- The perlocutionary act, which describes the effect of the act upon the listener.

Under these broad headings Prutting details examples which can be entered into the protocol (Prutting and Kirchner, 1983). This protocol is directed mainly for use with older children, but it does include some discussion of its application both to developmental stages and to children with language disorders.

Lund and Duchan (1983) also include a pragmatics assessment. Although the contextual element is implicit in any analysis of pragmatics, these authors lay great stress upon this aspect and their suggested protocol that is also arranged in four areas includes the following:

1. Situational context.
2. Intentional context.
3. Listener context.
4. Linguistic context.

Lund and Duchan provide detailed descriptions of each of these headings with examples of behaviours that may be subsumed under them.

None of these protocols includes procedures for eliciting behaviours. A procedure that does, is that of Blank and Marquis (1987), which is not standardised but individual educational plans can be drawn up from it.

Dewart and Summers' (1988) *Pragmatics Profile of Early Communication Skills* provides a descriptive and qualitative assessment of the child's functional communication. It is based on a structured interview with the parent or care-giver. Dewart and Summers state that the responses obtained can then be used as a basis for planning intervention. One criticism that has been levelled at this assessment though is that of Letts and Reid (1994), who say that because the test concentrates on 'normal' behaviours there is no room for the atypical. They and Bishop and Adams (1989) recommend individual profiling methods with the use of specific probes. By utilising 'discourse analysis' (which uses a preset coding) and/or 'conversation analysis' (where behaviours are not prescribed) it is possible to isolate problematic areas and then move on to test them more specifically.

A formal assessment of pragmatic skill, which is used more in the USA, is the Shulman Test of Pragmatic Skills (1985). It uses such probes with puppets eliciting behaviours from the children in different play contexts. Another standardised assessment that looks at children's ability to retell a narrative and can give insights into children's pragmatic abilities, is the Bus Story (Renfrew, 1972b).

Although this section has described the assessment of pragmatics as a separate element of communication its close relationship to semantics makes a separate delineation difficult. Bloom and Lahey's (1978) intersecting circles of form, content and use emphasise this. Additionally Smith and Leinonen (1992) discuss the need to assess the whole communicative event, not just the speaker's part in it. For instance Conti-Ramsden and Dykins (1991) discuss the effects of different listener styles on children in conversation and Panagos et al. (1988) and Gardner (1994) consider the possible influences of the speech and language therapy process itself.

Comprehension

Comprehension subsumes all other aspects of language. It involves the reception of phonological, grammatical and semantic information through sensory channels and its central integration, comparison and storage with past linguistic experience. Assessment of comprehension without reference to language production poses many problems and, in any case, the wisdom of such a strategy is debatable. If, as has been maintained throughout this text, language disorders are seen to be on a continuum of severity, then the imposition of an artificial dichotomy between receptive language on the one hand and production on the other, will hardly be conducive to effective remediation. Well-documented research has shown that those disorders where receptive problems predominate tend to include production deficits as well (Eisenson, 1972, 1985). Conversely where expressive problems are salient, it is comparatively rare not to find some degree of associated comprehension difficulty (Bishop, 1979; Adams, 1990). The exceptions may be cases diagnosed as dysarthrias or verbal dyspraxias. Prelinguistic development is as important as linguistic and procedures such as Gerard (1986) and Dewart and Summers (1988) deal with this.

Attention

Reynell (1969) considered that the development of fully integrated attention was an essential substructure of comprehension. This was measured on an observational developmental scale ranging from simple single channel through to fully integrated multimodal attention, which it is claimed is achieved by around 5 years of age (Cooper, Moodley and Reynell, 1978).

Auditory perception

Evidence regarding the precise role played by auditory perception is conflicting. Some researchers regard impaired auditory perception as one of the principal contributory features of severe language disorders (see Chapter 4). Traditionally the components of auditory perception that are examined are auditory discrimination, auditory sequencing and auditory memory. Importantly assessment of these areas have been further developed to cover aspects of linguistic and 'metalinguistic' word manipulation skills that are thought to underlay language and reading acquisition. These skills include word segmentation, rhyming judgements etc. (see Williams and Chiat, 1993; Stackhouse and Wells, 1993). Programmes such as the Nuffield dyspraxia assessment now carry material relating to such skills (Williams and Corrin, 1995).

Auditory discrimination

Most of the auditory discrimination tests currently in use are based on word recognition. The child can be required to differentiate between two 'minimal pair' words on a same/different basis (Wepman Auditory Discrimination Test) and the somewhat worrying feature of this test is the strong element of chance that the child will hit upon the right response (50%). To minimise this factor Morgan-Barry (1988) produced a Test of Auditory Discrimination and Attention, which requires the child to select the stimulus word presented by the therapist from a choice of two minimal pair pictures over three to six repetitions. A greater selection, a choice of three or four others, some of which are also minimally paired occur in the Renfrew Auditory Discrimination Test (Renfrew, 1972a).

Berry (1980) discusses the problems inherent in the assessment of auditory perception as the processes that underlie the discrimination of sustained on-going speech are likely to be different from those that are effective for discrimination of isolated sounds. Locke (1980) reviews currently prevailing methods of assessing auditory perception and suggests criteria that should be met to avoid the shortcomings that he regards as endemic in these, for example a need to observe context sensitivity, i.e. that phonemes should be placed in identical phonetic environments for both perception and production.

In a discrimination task, it is pointed out that there is a requirement to compare a sound just heard and stored in short-term memory with that in lexical long-term memory storage. This latter represents a composite of the sound that has been perceived on many different occasions and produced by many different people. To test the child's metaphonological awareness at this level it is possible to do rhyming judgements where pictures are provided but the words are not spoken by the tester. Therefore the child has to rely entirely on internal representations. Obviously the fact that the child can use their knowledge of real words for support can hide some subtle perceptual difficulties. A way round this is to use non-word stimuli and this has found to be diagnostically useful, for instance in dyspraxia (Bridgeman and Snowling, 1988) where non-word discrimination (of clusters) was poorer than real-word.

As Locke states: 'the clinical challenge is to separate the child who cannot detect a difference between two sounds from the child who detects a difference but considers it linguistically unimportant' (p. 456). In the first case, perceptual training may be indicated; in the second, there may be a need for phonological reorganisation.

Auditory memory and sequencing

There are two considerations that are of importance in assessment of temporal features. The first is the rate at which the child is able to process the incoming information and the second his ability to reproduce it in the correct order. Stark, Tallal and Mellits (1985) have reviewed experimental work, much of it their own, which considers the relationship between auditory temporal factors and receptive speech. Their view is that children with specific language disability have difficulty in processing rapid incoming information. When the acoustic transition was less than 40 msec duration language-impaired children failed to discriminate, but when the duration was increased to 80 msec they were successful. Tests of auditory sequencing such as the subtest in the ITPA recommend an interval between digits. But it is important to bear in mind that the time factor may be one cause of poor performance. This test requires the subject to repeat the sequence of digits. Referring back to the model of processing it is equally possible that failure may be the result of encoding problems and not of input.

Limitations of auditory memory have also been cited as being contributory to effective comprehension of language. The most usual way of assessing this is to get the child to repeat sentences of increasing length. There are differences between assessment that requires repetition of isolated words or strings of digits and those that rely on sentence repetition. In the latter case, performance is likely to be better, for the child will be able to make use of semantic cues.

Syntactic comprehension

Tests of syntactic comprehension were devised in response to a need for more specific diagnostic assessments that can pinpoint more precisely the areas of weakness that children have. It has already been pointed out that assessments such as the RDLS do not give any indication as to why a child has failed a certain item. Specific areas of syntactic failure, such as an inability to cope with indirect sentence forms have been strongly linked theoretically to SLI compared with younger normal children's performance (for details see Adams, 1990; Van der Lely and Harris, 1990; Bishop, 1992b; Van der Lely, 1994).

The assessment of grammar most widely in use currently is the TROG (Bishop, 1983) (and to a lesser extent TACL-R; Carrow-Wolfolk, 1985). It covers a range of grammatical and morphological structures that the subject identifies from a selection of pictures in response to a spoken stimulus. Wiig has written extensively on the assessment of language within a cognitive processing framework and her CELF-R assessment (1987) covers some areas of syntactic comprehension. The UK version (Semel, Wiig and Secord, 1987) of this has proved a useful addition to the clinic battery. Importantly the needs of ethnic minorities in this country are now being recognised and some English tests are now produced in other languages. For instance the Sentence Comprehension Test (Wheldall, Mittler and Hobsbaum, 1987) now has a Punjabi version.

Language production

Turning to language production, not unexpectedly there is somewhat less confusion, for at least here observable behaviour is being described. Assessment methods have evolved from standardised tests (e.g. Action Picture Test; Renfrew, 1988) has long been popular as a screening test of grammar and content) through to profiling procedures that are currently more favoured. Such profiles are derived from the transcription of language samples obtained from naturalistic observation or from elicited methods. With the increasing use of profiles, there has been a move away from equating results with specific language ages. Rather, they are interpreted as representing particular stages in language production. Crystal, Fletcher and Garman (1976) delineated seven such stages of syntactic development. The original version had been modified by 1982 in some respects (see note in Crystal, 1982b, for details, and Crystal, Fletcher and Garman, 1989).

The interdependence of the levels of language production is implicit in the profiles developed by a number of workers, such as the Bristol Developmental Language Scales and Crystal (1987) has more recently acknowledged the importance of considering language in an interactive framework and acknowledges the problems that are sometimes apparent in isolating a factor such as syntax. Miller (1981) discusses procedures for analysing speech samples. Among general analyses he includes MLU (Brown, 1973). For this, the mean number of words or morphemes is counted for each tone-group and the mean is computed for 100 such utterances. The resulting figure is then assigned to a stage that corresponds to a predicted developmental age. The measure is still frequently cited in research studies, but its reliability is open to question. Length of utterance does not of itself tell us much about its structure and is therefore not particularly useful as a prelude to remediation. A very short MLU may arise for reasons other than linguistic deficit. For example, because of respiratory restrictions, a dysarthric child may well produce truncated tone-groups. In 1987, Miller noted that an MLU matching strategy, whilst focusing on developmental change, limits the way in which language disability may be described.

Lexical retrieval

German (1985, 1987) has carried out considerable research in this field. Her protocol relies on naming of geometric shapes, colours, etc. and is intended for children aged 5;0–10;0 years. Her assessments were based on the protocol devised by Wiig and Semel (1984) since modified and included in the CELF assessment. In any such test it is important to differentiate between recognition and retrieval. Failure may be the outcome of either of these processes. The Test for Language Competence (TLC) also incorporates this area (Wiig and Secord, 1989) and covers the range 5–18 years, although this is probably less used in this country. Snyder and Godley (1992) point out, however, that it is often the strategies that children use to circumvent their difficulty, such as silence, circumlocution and fillers, which are as much of communicative interest as the problem itself. Only careful discourse or conversation analysis will reveal these subtleties.

Prosodic features

It is interesting to note that in the taxonomy of measurement he proposes, Miller includes many non-segmental features. All too often assessment procedures either overlook these or tack them on the end as a sort of afterthought, so that they then tend to receive only cursory attention. This does not make linguistic sense, for it is generally acknowledged that in the hierarchy of development, prosody precedes segmental phonology both in comprehension and production. Crystal (1982b) has devised a prosodic profile (PROP) which is valuable as an indicator for intervention. It requires the transcription into tone units of about 100 utterances. These are analysed on LARSP principles into clause, phrase and word types. The location of the nuclear tone (tonicity) and the pitch direction (tone) are noted. PROP is concerned mainly with intonational aspects of prosody. It is useful, however, to assess other features such as rate, pause and contrastive stress. This can be done on a qualitative basis. The importance of this is particularly apparent in the case of analysis of a phonological/ syntactic disorder. It must be emphasised that because there is so little research data available on the development of prosody, other than for intonation (e.g. Allen and Hawkins, 1978), it is not advisable to ascribe a developmental age to these tasks. Crystal (1987), referring to Medical Research Council study that he undertook, reported that prosodic impairment proved to be the most significant discriminating feature in a group of 30 language-handicapped children.

More recently, using the method of conversation analysis, Wells and Local (1993) have advocated the production of individual child profiles that take into account the interactional outcome of their prosodic idiosyncrasies. Their interesting paper clearly provides useful indications for the initiation of therapy.

Semantic features

If assessment of syntax presents problems because of an insubstantial theoretical base (Miller, 1987), these are even more apparent in the case of semantic assessment. In part this is due to the inherent difficulties in analysing the constituents of 'meaning', which by tradition have such strong philosophical connotations. In his description of the underlying theory, Crystal (1981) cautions against the common confusion that exists between comprehension and semantics. A comprehension test is not a semantic analysis, though semantic features may form a part of it.

His profile PRISM, (Crystal, 1982b) is subdivided into two sections; PRISM-G comprises semantic–grammatical items whilst PRISM-L categorises semantic–lexical features. The latter covers 16 pages and is an attempt to provide an inventory of the possible range of lexical fields that might be covered by teachers and therapists with children. It is noted that in order to obtain a representative sample, elicitation tasks will need to be undertaken in addition to that obtained from spontaneous speech. A study of the theoretical basis and of the profiling technique, leaves the reader not a little daunted by the complexities of the analysis and in particular of the interpretation of some of the items in the lexical section.

Aldred (1983) carried out an interesting small study of intervention in which she used PRISM as part of her assessment procedure. Her group of six children of age range 3;1–4;10 years divided into those with predominantly expressive problems and those with receptive difficulties. The 'expressive' group was characterised by a heavy reliance on clause structures, semantically high in content with a preponderance of information loaded lexemes: 'read books. Play train'. In contrast, the predominantly 'receptive' group revealed restricted semantic functions. There was a high proportion of spontaneous to responsive utterances, over-use of coordination, tag questions and stereotypes: 'home in there, it down and out'. Aldred concludes that, taken in conjunction with other assessments of pragmatics and structure, PRISM has good potential for delineating subgroups of language disorder. PRISM-L has undergone a critical evaluation and modification process (Long and Hand,1996). The evaluation of profiling techniques for incorporation into therapeutic programmes is an under-developed area of research, especially in such an area as lexical semantics.

Assessment of early expressive vocabulary is a procedure that has found favour with some researchers. It is certainly an easier method although the results lack the depth found in the semantic analyses described above. Locke (1985) includes a first-words assessment in her Living Language programme. This is a 100-word vocabulary list that includes nouns, verbs, prepositions and adjectives in that order. There is a wide variation among children who are developing language along normal lines and for this reason she sets a surprisingly low baseline of 10 words at 2;0 years. This scheme emphasises the use of vocabulary with less focus on how meaningful is its use. A situation familiar to most clinicians is that in which the child has been taught a vocabulary list by well intentioned parents. These are in effect labels with little regard to relational meaning.

Phonology

One of the most widely used phonological profiles in current use is PACS developed by Grunwell (1985). This is based on a contrastive analysis of elicited speech with options for further different types of analysis. Potentially it offers a very detailed, rather time consuming, breakdown of a child's phonological system.

In commenting on the realities of undertaking such detailed assessments, it is not our intention to minimise in any way their value. On the contrary, they are very rewarding in that they provide a direct line to plans for remediation. Furthermore they add information which strengthens the evidence for delineation of subgroups. Grunwell has suggested parallels between phonological development and the stages of syntactic development proposed by Crystal, Fletcher and Garman. She rightly cautions, however, as indeed do others, against a too rigid regard for age norms.

A disadvantage of many phonological assessments is that they are based on single-word samples. Crystal's PROPH does allow for the analysis of connected speech though this is not obligatory. An interesting clinical analysis that moves away from this is the work of Wells (1994) who has looked at across-word boundary phonology and shown how important this is for intelligibility. His framework is useful both for assessment and treatment ideas. An example of the limitations of single word sampling was apparent in a case study described by Morgan-Barry (1988) in which data using the PACS stimulus words, and that obtained from spontaneous speech yielded differing patterns. Probably a sample of ongoing speech plus an elicited sample offers the most reliable evidence.

Having found the patterns of phonological error that a child is making it is possible to carry out further investigations to isolate the areas of deficit that underly the problem. As Stackhouse and Wells point out, an error may occur because the child has an inaccurate internal phonological representation or accesses an inappropriate one. There may be a correct internal representation but the child realises it inaccurately. The comparison of spontaneous and imitative productions can reveal problems with output processing.

Other metalinguistic skills underlying language and phonology disorder can be assessed, such as rhyming and non-word repetition (which isolates articulatory ability divorced from lexical representations) as they may provide pointers for the most efficacious approach to remediation and are critical for reading development.

Accountability

Our concern throughout this chapter has focused on the need to provide the optimum conditions and opportunity for the investigation of the child's behaviour so that appropriate remediation may follow as a natural corollary. It is also necessary to consider the issue of accountability particularly with reference to evaluation of such remediation, for all clinicians have an obligation to ensure that to the best of their ability they are providing an appropriate service both to the children they treat and to the authorities that employ them (see Chapter 3).

In its narrowest sense, accountability requires an unwarranted measuring of work carried out. Siegel, Katsuki and Potechin (1985) observe that value questions arise continuously. Concern about which clients we should serve, what the criteria should be for accountability, how to measure the cost of services against the quality of life of clients. This last factor is particularly relevant and is one that seems to be at variance with the less acceptable facets of accountability. That changes in human behaviour cannot be so easily numerically recorded is to state the obvious and language presents a particularly complex field of behaviour. Efficacy studies of acquired language disorder have yielded disappointing results in terms of quantifying the value of therapy, but enlightened discussion has cautioned against taking such figures at their face value. Weakness of design and a multiplicity of variables has confused the findings. Additionally, as we have sought to emphasise, communicative ability adds up to more than a set of language scores (see Chapter 8). A broader definition of accountability is described by Douglass (1983). Legislative aspects are discussed, but he goes on to say that accountability requires a personal commitment on the part of the clinician to justify the quality of the service he or she offers to the person with a communication handicap.

Chapter 7
The nature and timing of intervention

Summary

This chapter discusses the principles underlying intervention and discusses the advantages and limitations of the range of facilities that is presently available including language units, special schools and routine health service provision. Comparison is made between statutory rights of language-disordered children in the UK and the USA. The subtypes of language disorder described in Chapter 5 are further considered with reference to appropriate types of intervention.

The management of children with developmental language disorders is dependent for its success on two overall factors:

- The presence of well trained and skilled professionals in all the relevant disciplines.
- Systems of health care and education that allow the expertise to be available to those who need it.

As has been noted throughout this text, the academic study of language disorders occurs in all the developed countries and many of the same types of investigations are carried out and conclusions reached. The principles of intervention derived from these conclusions are also common to a number of different nations. Were it not so, the study of language disorders in developing children would have little validity because the conditions described could only be related to individual cases. Where we see differences, they are of application and emphasis. Nevertheless, the service provision is basic to the philosophies and attitudes of professionals involved because one generation creates it and subsequent generations are influenced by it. This commonality is particularly important for colleagues within the European Union, as the Royal College of Speech and Language Therapists (RCSLT) liaises with professional bodies across the Union, with the aim of setting up pan-European standards of education and professional practice.

Whilst emphasising shared experience, within systems of health care among developed nations, however, we find considerable differences, although there is an overall trend towards early identification of and treatment for all developmental disabilities. Within the field of education there is also a common leaning that is having important consequences for those with language disorders. This is the integration of handicapped children into regular schools.

The philosophy of integration is unexceptionable because it aims to allow all children to participate fully in the life of the community and not to suffer isolation or stigma through disability. The practice can, however, be very penalising to those very children it purports to help. Integration of the handicapped depends for its success on excellent support services. These kinds of services are extremely vulnerable to economic cuts. We must view with alarm, therefore, any attempt to integrate children with special needs into regular schools at a time when the education system is starved of money and resources. Our language-disordered children are particularly vulnerable because we have not yet developed enough good techniques of remediation to propagate them with assurance. We still need time to examine how language-disordered children respond to specific management strategies and this cannot be done if the children are struggling to survive.

Since the first edition of this book was published, the National Curriculum has taken a foothold in England and Wales. There is concern as to the extent to which this prevailing wind will be tempered to the shorn lamb. Because children with language disorders lack the ability to integrate their language skills and place them at the benefit of further learning, they may forever be running into particular problems of comprehension and execution. Not all their skills will be retarded to the same degree, but the extent to which learning is affected cannot always be anticipated. The need of those with language disorders is for flexible provision that can cover structured language teaching as well as other educational measures. Flexibility is also needed in the timing of educational procedures and this is where the National Curriculum presents some problems (despite the fact that exemptions may be made for children within the Curriculum framework). We must therefore continue to propagate the need for special language units (attached to mainstream schools) where children can be given intensive help and where techniques of therapy and teaching can be developed and tested. It will probably always be necessary to retain a few residential special schools for those children whose problems are so profound that they need protection from the demands of the normal community until they have developed some learning strategies together with sufficient insight and maturity for survival. Protected communities are also necessary for children with severe medical problems or conditions that require a particular combination of medical, educational and social surveillance. Our existing facilities include individual therapy, remedial teaching, language unit placement and placement within a special school for children with disorders of communication. These facilities operate on the assumption that children who have failed to develop language in the normal way can be taught the sequence of abilities that should have developed spontaneously. They also operate upon the assumption that children can be trained to compensate for impaired language skills. A further assumption is that language-disordered children are penalised by society and so society owes them some special care in exchange. We do not propose to challenge this third assumption but the first two will be discussed.

Can language be taught?

This is a question posed by Harris (1984) in an essay that goes right to the heart of the matter. Harris argues that teaching and traditional forms of language intervention are incompatible with the development of natural language abilities in language-disordered children. Thus, interventionists should concentrate upon facilitating development and 'then document the emergence of each child's personal language curriculum' (p 249). If we are to stimulate language along normal lines, our success must depend on the extent to which we can stimulate the children to behave like normal language users. Unless the child can take over the language learning in a very active way, we can do little more than give a set of linguistic structures and as much communicative success as we can muster. Some children are going to be able to contribute more actively to language learning than others, not just by the virtue of temperament and intelligence, but because of the underlying nature of the disorder. The more impaired are those areas underlying comprehension, semantic and pragmatic skills, the more likely the child is to be perpetually restricted in language because he is not able to make language discoveries.

We have to accept that there are only some aspects of language that can be explicitly taught whether by capitalising on the skills of the mother or by later involving the child in a scientifically based and explicitly principled teaching programme. Language is characterised by structure and creativity. The basic rules have to be mastered in order that it can become the tool for communication, the expression of thought and all sorts of imaginative enterprises. The child needs to know his language and be able to reflect upon it. Normally developing children, having mastered the basic language structures and processes, will use them in all sorts of communal as well as individual activities. The pursuit of these activities will stimulate more variety of language forms. For example, young children coming together in pretend play will use politeness forms and verbal reasoning requiring a higher level of performance than is encountered among other exchanges (Garvey and Kramer, 1988). They are constantly stretching themselves cognitively and linguistically in the attempt to achieve together those goals that would be impossible apart. Their language development is not being stimulated by goals set by other people but by their own needs and interests.

Language teachers and therapists have recognised that natural situations, or those situations that occur naturally during the development of normal children, are necessary to stimulate normal language growth (Adams and Conti-Ramsden, 1995). This is very evident in the shift of remedial approaches from the modification of behaviour to the promotion of interaction. It is not useful to attempt to graft language structures or even language strategies on to an organism that is not receptive to new experiences. The difficulty was first perceived as one of generalisation. Individual components of language could be taught, but the difficulty lay in getting the child to make use of the components in his normal behaviour and to integrate them into a developing language system. The feasibility of helping language development through specified periods of intervention in a clinical setting has been severely questioned. Speech and language therapists are particularly vulnerable to such criticism because this is the way so many of them work. We may wonder, however, whether the individual clinician, working interactively with a young child in the presence of his mother, is more or less likely to achieve some gains in language growth than is the person who administers a specific training programme to a group of children in a class, even if it is administered every day. On the evidence of changes in test scores after a period of 18 months, the study of Edwards et al. (1984) found no significant difference in progress between group (intensive language class) therapy and individual treatment. These results, however, are qualified by (1) small numbers and (2) no control over the type of therapy given in these settings. It can be said, however, that it is unlikely to be the setting that dictates the effectiveness of the language therapy, but the extent to which this therapy can stimulate language learning in the child. Each facility must have a use. What is needed are good selection criteria or very good reasons for a child being given a particular type of intervention by a particular person in a particular place.

Effective intervention

Reviews of intervention approaches and discussions as to their success emphasise the importance of selecting the approach that is most appropriate for the individual case. Leonard (1981), writing about a number of approaches then current, found several to be effective when used appropriately, suggesting that their value was relative rather than absolute. Effective intervention resulted in language gains and had cumulative learning effects. Intervention approaches included:

- imitation based approaches;
- expansion approaches;
- focused stimulation approaches; and
- general stimulation approaches.

Fey (1986) discusses the whole process of language intervention, citing different approaches used in the accomplishment of different goals. For example, in training content–form interactions there are trainer-oriented approaches, child-oriented approaches and hybrid approaches. If the goal is to facilitate responsiveness to a conversational partner there are operant approaches, a number of which Fey specifies and child-oriented approaches as previously described by the author. Fey sees intervention as employing a range of procedures. These procedures are brought into being by an agent (clinician, teacher, parent) who 'stimulates or responds to a child in a manner that is consciously designed to facilitate development in areas of communication ability that are viewed as being at risk of impairment' (p. 40). Fey, in using this definition, accepts that a variety of approaches will be used by clinicians operating under markedly different conditions and with differing theoretical orientations. Because there is such a number of alternatives among intervention procedures, it is not easy to select the right one in every case. Perhaps it is even more important to avoid the wrong one. Kirk, on the subject of written language in 1983, makes a point that is also applicable to spoken language. If instruction is faulty, it may actively impede the learning of children whose preparatory skills are inadequate or barely adequate. To use a very simple illustration, if we choose a delayed speaker aged 3 years or so, who is just starting to use words referentially and try to take him through babbling procedures to improve his motor control, we are likely to impede his language learning adversely. On the other hand if we continue to encourage points and grunts with no attempt at articulatory shaping, we are not helping the child to achieve conventional utterances. Intervention is therefore all about *decisions*. We are particularly aware of this with the younger children because of the possibility of doing harm through not appreciating the nature of the emerging problem. Whilst it is possible to do harm at any age, we have less excuse when the child is older with more signs to offer us as to his needs.

When we select children for intervention, we must believe that our timing is right as well as our procedures appropriate. This applies at a number of different stages. The first decision is whether to intervene or to wait. The next may be to decide how intensively to intervene. If the child is very young, should our procedures be home based or centre based? If the child is older, should he or she attend a unit or a class for the language disordered? Unfortunately, some of these questions remain academic because there may be so few treatment possibilities open to the child. This concentrates decisions about selection. Which children should receive the benefits of our sparse resources? The information available from current outcome studies implies that it is the presence of the older language-impaired child, whose needs are well established and the persistent nature of these needs, which should dictate prioritisation. If we could identify who these children are in the early years and distinguish them from the language-delayed child, then we would be in a better position to reflect upon the usefulness of therapy (Enderby and Emerson, 1995). Fey, Catts and Larrivee (1995) state that 'it may be far more productive to view language impairment in preschoolers not only for what it is at present, but also for what it is likely to become as the child gets older' (p. 3).

Therapeutic and educational provision for language-impaired children

Since the passing of the 1981 Education Act, each local education authority (LEA) has a duty to ensure that special education provision is made for pupils who have special educational needs. This applies to children aged 2;0–19;0 years. When a child is perceived to be in need of special provision, the LEA must arrange for a comprehensive assessment to be carried out. This assessment must be multi-disciplinary and take account of both educational and medical factors together with input from the child's parents and the psychologist. Any written advice that arises from the assessment becomes a Statement of Special Educational Need. The LEA has a legal obligation to meet this need. Where provision within the normal school is agreed to be adequate, the formal statement may be waived. This means that the child can potentially participate in the provisions of the National Curriculum. Wedell (1980), writing about the application of the National Curriculum to children with special needs, makes the point that in teaching pupils with a wide range of abilities, teachers need to 'match the breadth of content at any one level of the curriculum to their pupils' capacity to cope with it'. He goes on to underline the need for such children to be able to focus on the content at one level, which is essential for the attainment of the next level. There is therefore a need for modification and flexibility in application. This is especially true where the learning difficulty includes language impairment.

A formal statement must be reviewed annually, whenever there is a change in circumstances or at the request of the parents. The situation has occurred many times where an assessment team has found a need for intensive speech-language therapy but the LEA is not in a position to provide it and the health authority cannot afford to do so, and despite recent changes the LEA can always claim lack of funds as a last resort to refuse a special placement. Many disputes have surfaced as a result of this lack of political will to assume responsibility for the finance of genuine need. For example the now famous 'Lancashire judgement' represents the ruling of the High Court in a case where a language-impaired child was not receiving the speech and language therapy his statement suggested he needed, due to the lack of provision of therapy in his local region. The Lancashire judgement stated that the LEA had a duty to provide that therapy. Since then financial considerations have been used as a loop-hole by LEAs to escape from this burden. A special needs tribunal system has now been set up to, hopefully, dispense with the necessity for parents to have to resort to court action for the law to be upheld. It cannot be overstated that the present unsatisfactory state of affairs in certain parts of the UK, in terms of special provision for language-impaired children, is a direct result of: (1) successive governments reneging on promises made in the Education Acts; and (2) a lack of public debate and concern on these issues, despite the efforts of bodies such as AFASIC and RCSLT to publicise the issues.

Revisions to the 1981 Act have clarified the position with regard to the position of speech and language therapy. However, there is considerable variation in different parts of the country. The College of Speech Therapists issued a position paper (1988b), which gives guidelines for speech and language therapists 'to ensure, as far as possible, that practices within their District allow for their full and appropriate involvement in the identification, assessment and meeting of Special Educational Needs'. It acknowledges that terminology may vary in different parts of the country but contends that general principles remain the same. *Communicating Quality*, the professional standards manual for speech and language therapists, also sets out guidelines for clinicians in this matter (College of Speech and Language Therapists, 1990).

Contrasting the British experience with that of the US is illuminating, and illustrative of the complexities of this debate. In the US the education authority or school district enters into a contract with the parents of the handicapped child to carry out an individualised education programme (IEP). This IEP is drawn up following multi-disciplinary assessment if necessary, and with the full agreement of the parents. If the programme as agreed by both parties is not carried out, parents may sue the school district. If they are successful, the district must provide the services. The IEP has thus much stronger backing than the British 'Statement' because it relates back to the Bill of Rights, via Public Law. It is a basic human right not to be discriminated against. Legal action is therefore the immediate recourse in the case of default. Whilst the system has a strength that many British parents campaigning for services must envy, it does lead to an almost intolerable amount of litigation, which can sour relations and slow down procedures. It can also lead to a certain amount of teaching to task because professionals having put their names to highly specified procedures do not feel free to take a more creative route, even if one presents itself. This can be a real detriment to dynamic language therapy.

One might wish to question strongly why there should be such widespread variation in provision for language-impaired children as exists currently in the UK. Provision varies across geographical and local authority boundaries, and the model of provision adopted appears to have less to do with the intervention requirements of the children than budgetary and ideological stances. The outcome of such manoeuvring is that some LEAs provide integrated education for language-disordered children, and some make special unit provision, whilst others (and they are in an increasingly small minority) are prepared to pay for residential places. The Education Act of 1993 entailed the preparation of the Code of Practice on the Identification and Assessment of Children with Special Educational Needs. The Code recommends strongly the education of all children with special needs within mainstream education. It is intended to provide guidelines for schools and LEAs in their provision for all children with special needs, including the language-impaired (Williams, 1996). Many schools now have special needs coordinators, who might function as a point of contact for an external speech and language therapist. The Code, despite representing a small step forward, cannot detract from the bare fact that there is insufficient speech and language therapy available to meet the needs of all children in school who require it, and that providing a 'helper' in a mainstream classroom for a language-impaired child cannot replace the expertise of a specialist teacher and therapist to whom the child should have access. Below we describe some of the specialist provision which is still available – but we do not know for how long.

Special schools for the language-impaired

These schools aim to deal intensively with the children's problems so that most transfer to mainstream education before school-leaving age. Children may be resident or day pupils, they may have receptive and/or expressive language problems, but they should be free from severe hearing impairment, generalised severe learning difficulties, childhood autism, severe emotional disturbance or severe physical handicap. Whereas children with these difficulties very frequently have language difficulties, it would be impossible for small schools to provide appropriate teaching and therapy for such a range of handicapping conditions. Such restrictions are common to special schools of this nature, not only in the UK, but also in the USA and in Australia (Ellis Robinson, 1987). It should be noted that there appears to be a pragmatic shift from exclusion criteria, to take into account the fact that children with severe speech and language impairments rarely present with such a pure diagnosis, but frequently have associated deficits in the social or cognitive domains.

Curricula for special schools and language units

The more closely the school pursues the aim of eventual integration of the children into mainstream schooling, the more closely must it adhere to the mainstream curriculum. It must therefore attempt to combine a wide and varied curriculum with specialised language teaching. The residential special schools may concentrate on a more specialised aspect with use of augmentative communication systems. Individual therapy is prescribed as well as the participation of the speech and language therapist in the language activities of the classroom. Although integration back into the regular school community is the aim of the special school, there are a number of other goals. These are set out in one school prospectus (Ewing School, Manchester, 1988) as follows:

- To develop in our pupils as full an understanding and use of language as possible. To give them confidence to use what language they have in the widest possible social context. For a few very handicapped individuals, this may mean encouraging skills in compensating for spoken language which may always be a difficult medium for them.
- To develop as far as possible the basic skills of reading, writing and number. Again for a few pupils this may well mean concentrated effort in learning what is absolutely essential for them for life beyond school.
- Inclusive of the first two points, the wider curriculum is aimed at helping pupils who remain through to school-leaving age to lead interesting and useful lives as members of the community; also to encourage the development of personal interests and advanced skills to the highest possible level of competence.

It was pointed out in our first chapter that those who encounter language-disordered children for the first time in a special school setting may receive a much more positive impression than they would if they were seeing individual children experiencing failure in the normal school. All special schools want to receive their pupils before they experience too much demoralisation through failure. Lea (1986), writing to this point, refers to the growing reluctance of some authorities to continue sending severely language-disordered children to residential special schools. This could be coincidental upon the mainstreaming philosophy and the lack of money for education and must therefore be viewed with suspicion. Lea does state, however, that if residential special schools are to campaign for candidates it is incumbent on them to keep abreast of modern thought, practice and technology and to develop and share expertise.

The move away from residential provision could be seen as a positive one if it meant that all LEAs were committed to setting up sufficient and appropriate language units within their schools. This is hardly the case, although provision is certainly improving and likely to continue.

Language units

The charitable organisations ICAN (Invalid Children's Aid Nationwide) and AFASIC (Association For All Speech Impaired Children) have issued guidelines for language units. ICAN's guidelines follow a survey carried out in 1987 (Hutt and Donlan) into provision. The guidelines ask a number of important questions that must be satisfactorily answered before a language unit should be established. They relate to type of handicap, availability of classroom and other space, involvement of head teacher and other staff of the school in which the unit is to be placed, availability of suitably qualified teaching staff or provision for training them, availability of a suitably qualified educational psychologist to be involved in admission and discharge procedures and also in general support. This preliminary thinking is related to the lack of overall direction in the setting up of language units, with each LEA having its own standards and determining its own criteria for the selection of both children and staff. The situation is exacerbated when the language unit is a joint venture between LEA and district health authority. Lack of uniformity is also a point made in the AFASIC guidelines which indicate, however, that LEAs are now seeking help in the setting up of language units and require examples of good practice. With the combined proselytising activities of AFASIC and ICAN, we may hope to see a more clearly defined and cohesive policy towards language unit provision. All recommendations suggest that language units should be attached to mainstream schools with provision for gradual integration and with opportunities to share as many activities as are feasible. Provision is recommended for children upwards of 3 years with priority being given to the age range 3;0–7;0 years by LEAs establishing units for the first time. Once criteria for infant and junior level provision are established, units should be set up in the middle school.

The ICAN guidelines recognise that many children with below average non-verbal ability also have specific language disorders. They therefore suggest that units for these children be established in schools for children with moderate learning difficulties.

The guidelines recognise that language impairment will be present in some degree where there is:

1. physical disability;
2. severe or moderate learning difficulty;
3. behavioural and/or other emotional problems;

4. hearing loss;
5. autism;
6. severe reading and spelling difficulty sometimes known as dyslexia;
7. other handicaps less frequently.

It is assumed that children suffering from these difficulties are allocated provision on the basis of their primary disability. Also excluded from language unit provision should be those children who are learning English as a second language and who do not have a primary (i.e. mother tongue) language disorder. These exclusions are in accord with the residential school directive and, in theory at least, are sound. Naturally where children with other handicaps are being severely penalised by language impairment, the position is more difficult to justify. Schools and units that exist specifically for the language-disordered must nevertheless use relatively stringent criteria or they will end up helping no one and providing nothing. But it is expedient to note that individual LEAs and speech and language therapy services may set their own admission criteria, which increasingly may allow children with autistic spectrum disorders, or even children with additional learning difficulties into a language unit. The decision for placements in an LEA will (hopefully) be made on the individual's needs and the provision available.

ICAN suggest another group that should be excluded and this leads to rather more problems. This is the comparatively large group of children with language delay arising from 'a minimum of linguistic demands being made during the preschool years'. In order for this criterion to be applied justly, the succeeding recommendations need to be followed very closely. These are: that the child be placed in a mainstream school that supplies a basic curriculum and, within this, that there should be extra group teaching from a support teacher. Identification should be made of areas that need enrichment and suitable experience and materials provided. The speech and language therapist should be available, either as a consultant or to give individual therapy as required. Where no such facilities exist for regular teacher/therapist consultation, these children will fare very poorly. Nevertheless the recommendation is correct. Children who are capable of learning language through general stimulation should not be placed in classes where the emphasis is upon compensatory strategies.

Finally, it is recommended that children with severe articulation problems arising from dysarthria alone should only be placed in language units if no alternative is available. The prognosis for these children is usually poor and so their long-term sojourn in a language unit could deprive children of the means whereby they could learn to master the language system and thus function effectively in mainstream school. Whilst the ruling is not questioned the terminology here is rather confused. Dysarthria is not solely an articulatory problem; indeed this may be secondary to other deficits of respiration and phonation. Language disorder is also likely concomitant. It seems likely too that, if there is such a severe neurogenic language disorder, there will be some degree of associated physical handicap that would place such a child within the aegis of a school for physically-handicapped children and where it is hoped they would receive appropriate teaching and speech and language therapy, including the provision of alternative forms of communication where necessary.

These considerations bring up the whole question of prognosis, which has a place in decision making, though exactly what that place is, is by no means clear. There are a number of children whose language disorders suggest a poor prognosis but who are entitled to help. We are not ready to exclude children from language therapy or teaching because of possible poor prognosis and it is to be hoped we never will be. Prognosis may reasonably affect the nature and aims of therapy and the site of delivery. Schery (1985) makes the point that remedial programmes should be modified to meet the needs of children who are not likely to make good progress. However, the list of predictive factors that Schery gives have not been widely agreed. They were the result of a large statistical study of language correlates that has been challenged on a number of grounds (Kahmi, 1985; Bishop, 1987a). Paul (1995) stresses the importance of accurate prognosis. If the prognosis is not fulfilled, then it may be because (a) intervention has been ineffective, or (b) the prognosis was incorrect (see Chapter 8).

Integration or separation: implications for provision of education from long-term outcome studies

Perhaps the most positive way to view the benefits of special education is to look at the long-term outcome for language-disordered children; not just in terms of later language performance, also with reference to later social and employment opportunities. After all, education is for life. Surprisingly, there are relatively few studies in the area.

Paul and Cohen (1984) reviewed a group of children with serious language disorders who had received full initial evaluations at an average age of 6;5 years. The average age of the 18 children seen at follow-up was 14;2 years. The subjects had originally been placed in two groups. One group consisted of children with development language disorders, but no social deficits. The other group was deemed 'atypical developmental language disorder' because the children showed social withdrawal, poor or fleeting social relations and some of the sensory and motor responses of autism. All subjects had previously been diagnosed as 'aphasic'. Paul and Cohen do not discuss their atypical group in relation to semantic–pragmatic language deficits. However, they do state that none of the children satisfied the full criteria for infantile autism. It is possible, however, that they resembled severe cases of semantic–pragmatic disorder.

These authors found that the children with developmental language disorder and a high non-verbal IQ had a better outcome than those with low non-verbal IQ in terms of language growth and educational function. They also state that receptive skill together with intellectual capacity seem to be more important determinants of school placement than is speech because children with good understanding can function in less restrictive settings even when their expressive skills are less advanced: 86% of the low IQ developmental disordered language group and all of the atypical group had found placement in highly restrictive special day or residential schools. Only 50% of the high IQ children with developmental language disorders had been placed outside regular schools. IQ appeared to account for a great deal of the differences among the groups. The low IQ children differed from the atypical group only in degree of communicative intent. The latter group remained seriously deficient in communication. Paul and Cohen therefore argue that deficiency in early social skills has prognostic value in relation to communication. However, because both the low IQ groups showed poor language outcome, social skills do not emerge as a strong predictor of language growth.

This study has obvious implications for those concerned with provision. Its findings lend support to the ICAN recommendation for language units to be set up in schools for slow learning children. When LEAs find that they have to choose between setting up units for one group or another, the implications are less clear. One argument suggests that children with good language prognosis should have the advantage of the best facilities available because they can benefit most and make a speedier return to mainstream school. Another argument is to give the most comprehensive and intensive help to children who may do poorly because they would not survive in any other situation. A very cogent point to make is that all members of staff working in schools or units where a comparatively small number of children are receiving intensive remediation, need to see progress. If only those children with a poor prognosis are admitted, or if children are admitted after the time when they might learn best, the burden upon professional staff and their aides is particularly heavy. Although there is a good deal to be said for separating slow moving from faster moving children, it is valuable for staff members to be able to work with both groups.

A further study by Stone (1992), followed up 59 young people who had previously attended a language unit in the UK. Of those traced the majority had moved from the language unit to mainstream education, whilst a substantial minority remained in special units. A significant proportion of past pupils did attain some basic technical qualifications and occasionally a formal academic one. Many, however, continued to need support from the family with basic literacy tasks, and it is of interest that many of the pupils themselves expressed a desire for continuing support from the speech and language therapist well into the adolescent years. It is notable that Stone reports a high degree of retrospective enthusiasm for special and separate education of the language-impaired child from the children themselves. She concludes (p. 307), 'children with severe speech and language disorders need early intensive speech therapy and/or early admission to a speech and language unit'. Support in the mainstream integrated setting is essential later in the child's life.

For integration of these children in mainstream education to be effective it must be actively resourced. This is the stark message to come out clearly from a case study by Marshman and Miller (1994). The child whom they followed into a regular classroom, although successful in some parts of the integration process, still required considerable help, especially with literacy skills well into the second year of the programme of integration. Teachers, although willing to help, already have enough duties to carry without being expected to squeeze more training into a long day. Therefore it is simply not sufficient to 'dump' language-impaired children into mainstream host classrooms. Their integration requires *continuing professional and financial support*, both for host school training and for ongoing specialist advice. The provision of both of these could be described at the present time as, at best, patchy. *This is the principal problem for the advancement of integration, and one that cannot denied by ideological posturing*.

Inclusion criteria and staffing

Language unit provision will generally be for cases of developmental language disorder though some of the much smaller number of acquired cases may be taken. These do not generally include children with Landau–Kleffner syndrome who may need more medical attention than can be provided in a unit. The Landau–Kleffner syndrome is one that is acquired somewhere between the ages of 2 and 5 years. The child will have developed language but will lose it progressively, starting with verbal comprehension. The effects of the loss of comprehension on the child may be such as to suggest that he is suffering from hearing loss or behavioural disturbance but the disorder is that of auditory receptive aphasia (Robinson, 1987). Children with Landau–Kleffner syndrome are likely to have seizures and EEG examinations will show abnormal and epileptic features. The prognosis is variable. Some children recover their language function whilst others show permanent impairment with or without further seizures. The children who fail to recover language spontaneously are likely to need a protected residential environment or one which is part of a neuropaediatric unit because of the severity of the disorder and its medical implications.

ICAN guidelines have taken the step of specifying the four broad groups of language-disordered children most suited to language unit placement:

- Children with phonological–grammatical problems. This group has been described in Chapter 5 as the phonological–syntactic group. These children are expected to constitute the majority of the language unit clientele.
- Children who have the above problems with the accompaniment of a receptive disorder. It is suggested that only one or two children with major comprehension problems be placed in each class.
- Children with semantic–pragmatic problems. It is suggested that only children with mild forms of this disorder be placed in units. Children with severe disorders would be better placed in a protected environment where integration with mainstream classes is not part of the programme
- Children with articulatory difficulties based upon impaired coordination of the fine movements required for speech.

It is recommended that one teacher and one therapist be appointed full time to a class within a language unit. A class should consist of six to eight children. In addition there should be an assistant to the teacher or therapist and, as a resource person, an educational psychologist with special experience in developmental language disorders. The provision of speech and language therapy is complicated by the fact that speech and language therapists have typically been employed by the Health Service following the recommendations of the Quirk committee in 1972. Thus they are not immediately at the disposal of the LEAs (save for some isolated individuals). This dichotomy affects language-disordered children at many levels. It can result in the failure to detect subtle language disorders among the school-aged population. It can also result in the provision prescribed in a child's statement of special need failing to be carried out because the statement concerns the child's education, and speech and language therapy is provided from the health service budget. Among the many factors that militate against an integrated service for the language-disordered child, this administrative division is outstanding. In some districts, the goodwill and exertions of professionals keep the problems to a minimum, but no combination of goodwill and exertion is proof against sheer lack of personnel.

Meeting the need

We must now look at how previous points about the nature of language disorders and the differentiation of clinical subtypes can be integrated into this discussion of the principles and practicalities of intervention. In discussion of how best to help the children, we must bear in mind that their level of attainment will be determined by the extent to which they are able to use their own resources to compensate for their deficiencies. 'The extent to which a child is motivated to use whatever limited abilities he has determines his degree of success' (Wedell, 1980). We believe that if the child is developing language in an aberrant way, or if he is severely delayed, he must receive language teaching that assists this compensation and motivates him as an individual. General programmes of language development or stimulation will not be adequate or appropriate. Compensation may be assisted by building up individual language strengths, thus helping the child to find his own language-learning strategy. Alternatively it may be promoted by working away at weak features in order to strengthen them and improve the whole performance.

Teaching to strength or to weakness is a matter for individual decision. It has been our experience that when the child's overall cognitive or intellectual level is not high, teaching to weakness may prove discouraging. There is not enough language matrix to support the weak skill, and battering away at it may cause breakdown in overall function. Working through strength is a good therapeutic principle and should only be jettisoned upon very special consideration. We have little evidence to show that repeated work on, for example, auditory memory, can improve the memory. Improvement is more likely to come about through a number of compensatory strategies that arise from insight and resource.

Because we are working with developing children we must expect that the natural processes of maturation will exert their influence. The factors contributing to the language disorder will, both individually and collectively or interactively show change. It is the object of early intervention to accelerate this maturation. We may also expect to see a shift in the pattern of the disorder both as a result of therapy and because of the natural progress of the condition.

The following cases illustrate this pattern shift:

S was referred at 3;10 with no spoken language. Hearing was normal and comprehension as tested on the RDLS and the Peabody Picture Vocabulary Scale was on a par with chronological age. Social interaction was normal and S both responded to and initiated communication. Her speech performance was restricted to emotive jargon in which only mid-vowels and glides were noted. The only consonants were /n/, a dental /d/ and an occasional bilabial fricative. Direct stimulation produced recognisable approximations for the consonants /p/ /b/ /d/ /k/ and /g/. S was unable to imitate a phonetic pattern and at first was also unable to imitate a vowel with intonation.

During therapy, S learned to imitate rising and falling cadences using sustained vowels. Articulatory shaping developed spontaneously during this time, but not the ability to imitate a phonetic sequence. Imitation of simple words consisting of CV combination only was achieved by 5 years. As the words were linked together by the coordinate 'and' (or a close approximation) a simple phonological system started to emerge. At 7 years, S was enrolled in a newly-opened language unit with the diagnosis of expressive aphasia, word-finding difficulty and severe articulation disorder. Her overall score on the WISC was 96, within normal range. At that time, abnormal prosody was still evident in utterances of more than three or four words. Normal prosody was demonstrated in short familiar phrases, e.g. 'I don't know'. Sequencing difficulties were still apparent during a demonstration session at 9;10 years when the unfamiliar word 'Jubilee' was rendered as 'julibill'; this was corrected only after several minutes of instruction. At that time pragmatic sophistication was apparent in the way S handled conversation, following leads, initiating and giving new information when appropriate. Comprehension difficulties were now apparent in complex linguistic constructions, but needed to be probed for. S was able to transfer into mainstream schooling with additional support from the speech and language therapist and educational psychologist. Her reading skills were sufficiently well established to allow her to develop pleasure in reading, albeit at a somewhat unsophisticated level.

Motor sequencing skills and overall motor performance showed more evidence of abnormality during and after an adolescent growth spurt. Socially, S tended to cling to her family and lacked assertiveness. Both social and motor skills improved considerably after a period at a residential college where she was able to receive regular physiotherapy. Residual problems centred upon spelling and pronunciation of words containing clusters consonants. There appeared to be a link here in that spelling still lacked phonetic underpinning.

During her development and through the help received in the language unit and elsewhere, S developed very obvious strategies to help maintain control of language. One was the recourse to scanning or abnormal prosody when essaying long utterances. By breaking up utterances into short tone units she may have been able to facilitate processing including the retrieval of phonological representations of content and function words. Striving to establish meaning was often accompanied by a regression in clarity of articulation. However, she was able to help herself by good pragmatic function. For example, after stumbling over the phrase 'physically handicapped' she said 'like in wheelchairs'. During her early years, S presented a picture of verbal apraxia. The following characteristics were evident:

1.   Impaired ability to imitate at word and at sound level.
2.   Impaired prosody.
3.   Impairment of motor planning and timing.
4.   Impairment of monitoring.
5.   Impaired ability to carry out a sequence of movement, particularly at speed.

Later she showed characteristics of phonological–syntactic syndrome:

1.   Lack of articles, prepositions and pronouns.
2.   Omission of word endings.
3.   Faulty articulation.
4.   More difficulty with comprehension of language than initial performance suggested.

It is likely that the apparent shift from one type of language disorder to another was predominantly associated with cortical reorganisation, but demands placed upon her and the support given by her environment promoted the use of language. The combination of these attributes associated with skilled teaching encouraged mastery of language form. A crucial therapeutic procedure was the setting up of the articulatory loop. This subsystem has been shown to be involved in subvocal rehearsal and associated with memory span (Hitch and Halliday, 1983).

The second case history also shows the shift in the main features of language disorder in a young female:

J was born normally to a mother who had been hospitalised for 6 months during pregnancy because of hyperemesis (acute vomiting). The child had a birth weight of 6lb 2oz. Early development appeared normal. Subsequently there was mild spasticity of the right leg and delayed and unintelligible speech which was exacerbated by dysarthria. There was also sequential difficulty at word and sound level. Speech and physiotherapy were started at 3 years of age. J was intelligible at 7;0 years, but a severe reading problem then became apparent. At 17 years of age, J a girl of strong character and good overall intelligence had come to the following conclusion, 'I feel that as I cannot read now, I never will'. However, following full investigation and the construction of a specially designed reading programme, some gains were made. The investigation carried out by a psychologist and a speech and language therapist showed problems of analysis and synthesis in sound patterns, affecting both speech and spelling though the latter skill was now more conspicuously abnormal. For example 'alphabetically' became 'alphurbatilly', 'told' was 'tal', 'plod' was 'plood' and 'dyslexia', 'dislects'. The speech and language therapist's report also draws attention to occasional word substitutions and recall difficulties. The psychologists found clear evidence of reading/spelling disorder aggravated by years of educational difficulties.

Writing of her life some 15 years later, she states, 'I don't have the inquisitive mind to pick up a piece of paper and see what is on it' and 'a book is just a load of print'. She has made the decision to avoid all reading as far as possible. And as an overall policy, 'I try to put myself in situations where I know I can cope well and avoid others' but 'I know I am very dependent on other people'. The sum of characteristics of this language disorder would place it in the phonological–syntactic syndrome group. However, the spasticity and articulatory difficulties place it towards the motor end of the spectrum. J would be one of those children with expressive difficulties allied to cerebral palsy, originally described by Morley. Initial therapy for such children tends to focus on movement control. In order to anticipate and so far as is possible prevent severe secondary disabilities, the ability to perceive and to analyse sound sequences should be promoted at the same time. The shift which took place in J's case was from a condition of mild cerebral palsy affecting the organisation of movement to a broader condition of perceptual and linguistic deficit. The programme of intervention was not sufficiently comprehensive to prevent the severe language problem affecting a number of skills.

Interestingly though J showed considerable resource in coping with her difficulties in the running of her life, she did not, either as a young child or subsequently, develop spontaneous strategies to assist herself in mastering sound patterns (for examples of such strategies, see Weeks, 1974). Her failure to do so might at first have been due to lack of awareness of her problems and later to discouragement as to her inability to surmount them. It is possible, but by no means certain, that more helpful self-help strategies could have been stimulated by a cohesive and comprehensive intervention programme. In noting the absence of such programmes in the past, however, we must also be aware of cases where they have been instituted and have still not been able to guard against the shift in the condition or the variety of its manifestations. Reference has already been made to the account given by Damico (1988). This case contradicts the unfortunately strong impression made by some observations, that early speech and language therapy may simply concentrate on polishing up the child's utterance and eliminating articulatory errors. In the case described by Damico, there was thorough investigation of the language disorder in a child of 5;11 years. The characteristics were syntactic and semantic problems which were tackled by regular and systematic language therapy. The case was assessed and reassessed (see Chapter 6) and discharge was only carried out when gains had been shown in all the areas of deficit. Six years later, the child was referred back to the language clinician exhibiting severe behavioural and communicative disorder. Investigation showed a number of abnormal language behaviours that had been insufficiently probed earlier.

Damico gives a number of interesting reasons for the failure of initial therapy to eliminate subsequent problems. The impression produced is one of an experienced and conscientious clinician who is limited by the procedures available to him at any one time. However, we could contend that there can be no absolute safeguards against the recurrence of a language disorder because even the most inspired clinician must be limited in what he can observe and predict. We can safeguard ourselves against myopic adherence to a limited approach and alert ourselves to the limitations of the prevailing viewpoint. Teachers and therapists who have worked with language-disordered children over a long period of time tend to adopt approaches described by one of us (BBB), as 'core implicit and crisis induced' (Byers Brown, 1982). Though assessment and observation will show the nature of the problems and intervention procedures are then designed to help the child to compensate. As we encourage the child to grow and experiment in language, different prob-lems or additional ones may be revealed. As we work hard with the chil-dren, we may push them to process more language elements than they can comfortably handle. There may then be regression in form or func-tion whilst reorganisation takes place. The therapist or teacher will support and encourage the child and family at times of crisis and if these periods are wisely handled further growth may result.

In developing children of otherwise good endowment, the limits of capacity and predictions of growth cannot be gauged to a nicety. Where limitations are general and profound, more protection and less pressure towards growth may be pursued. Failure to create appropriate effort in any handicapped child is likely to lead to passivity and inertia. It is possible that some of our early approaches to language intervention may have contributed to this result in the past by too little emphasis on func-tion and interaction and too much emphasis on form. It will be inter-esting to see whether young language-disordered children can take on a more active, dynamic role in subsequent language teaching if they are prepared for it on the lines indicated by Aldred (1983). In this article a language group within the nursery environment is described. Emphasis throughout the activities was placed upon language in context and use. The natural social environment of the group was seen as the stimulator of language interactions with natural reinforcement being provided for successful use. The children admitted to the group received comprehen-sive individual assessments including analysis of a 30-minute speech sample through the LARSP and PRISM procedures (see Chapter 6).

Phonology was analysed through the Grunwell model (1975) and the language functions outlined by Halliday (1975) were used as the framework for describing language use.

The children demonstrated delay in all parameters of language development. Two groups could be identified, one with predominant deficit in verbal expressive abilities and one with predominantly poor verbal receptive skills. The expressive group showed initially poor grasp of phrase structure with relatively advanced clause structure high in semantic content and relying upon information-loaded lexemes. Phonology was delayed. The receptive group showed advanced phrase structures, stereotyped clause structures and restricted semantic functions. This group showed a few phonological immaturities. Children in both groups showed gains following intervention. The expressive group added to their range of linguistic structures and the receptively-impaired group improved in interpersonal communication and in the regulatory aspects of language function. All children advanced in verbal receptive skills. Aldred comments that perhaps the most important change was in their social-communication skills. The children widened the functional range of their language and actively sought to widen their own environment. This change came about through therapy, which aimed to follow the child's lead, and which relied upon the social interaction developed in the group to provide the primary motivator. Parents were actively involved and became increasingly aware of the functions of language. As a natural consequence, they started to give their children increased communicative responsibility in the home. This type of management would appear to have a great deal to offer to the preschool child. It stimulates language development in a way that leaves parent and child with functional gains. It could thus provide a valuable precursor to individual therapy or to language unit placement and special teaching.

Intervention procedures in relation to specified clinical subtypes

In our discussion of intervention procedures we will follow the order indicated by our language processing model in Chapter 4.

Verbal auditory agnosia

Because this condition is characterised by inability to interpret information presented through the auditory channel, the thrust of the intervention procedure should be through the visual channel. Children who have severe auditory perceptual problems, or who show the full syndrome of verbal auditory agnosia (receptive aphasia), are candidates for special school placement. This is true for both the developmental syndrome and for the condition acquired in early childhood (Landau–Kleffner syndrome). The psychological picture is different in the acquired cases because, if children have started to make sense of the speech around them, the sudden loss of this ability will be very frightening and bewildering.

Young children may first be enrolled in individual therapy programmes whilst suitable educational placement is found for them. The therapist may then institute a signed system of communication, which will be the basis of the child's acquisition of language structure. Several special schools in Britain have adopted the Paget–Gorman signing system and so speech and language therapists will use this with individual children who later may be offered places in these schools. Signing provides an interim measure to promote communication and lay down word order concept in children with less severe impairment. The Paget–Gorman signing system has been described as an important means of cueing some children in to the spoken and written word and to the conventions of word order for it is a grammatically-based system. A useful paper on the need to establish criteria of measurement in signing systems is that by Faucett and Clibbons (1983). The acquisition of signing allows aphasic adolescents to share social activities with the signing deaf, thus enlarging their circle of friends. Because they are inevitably isolated from their normal peer groups, this enlargement is important. The restrictions that the condition imposes upon their cognitive and social development means that they may remain immature and egocentric. Social contacts, shared activities with normal children and the promotion of team efforts form a very large part of the schools' activities.

The first programme to help these children was developed by McGinnis (1963); it became established as 'the association method'. Subsequently criticised for its rigidity, it was replaced by several schemes that employed visual representations, e.g. Lea's Colour Pattern Scheme (Lea, 1965) to teach parts of speech and word order. Whereas the McGinnis method placed emphasis on visual representation of single sounds in order to facilitate utterance, the Lea method taught whole words. This enabled children to move on to simple written language as a means of communication whilst they were still unable to produce intelligible words. The question as to whether to try to generate utterance at the same time as teaching symbol representation through the visual form was in most cases influenced by the population within the various establishments. It was deemed very unlikely that some children would ever be able to produce intelligible utterances and so speech would be of no practical value to them. We now know that this is not necessarily the case and that for some children there is a better prognosis. Early intervention should therefore include auditory and articulatory training in a sequence of stages (Vance, 1991), at least as an exploratory phase. The principle of employing visual modality methods to compensate for auditory deficits has not changed. A means must be provided that will lead to the acquisition and storage of lexical items and grammatical structures, and this is likely to be through the visual modality.

Rapin and Allen point out that the population of children with verbal auditory agnosia will include children who have autistic features and are profoundly retarded intellectually. Such children are unable to acquire language through a grammatically-based signing system, though they may fare better with an iconic method like MAKATON. In their discussion of auditory agnosia, Rapin and Allen subscribe to the view that this receptive syndrome (without autism) is a 'pure' syndrome with severe consequences for language processing including production. We would agree with this view because these children suffer by order of magnitude when compared with those who have comprehension difficulties when faced with continuous language. The children with verbal auditory agnosia do not understand some auditory sequences and misunderstand others. The auditory channel may not useful to them as a means of learning. Fortunately, the condition is rare. However, our discussion of language-processing models draws attention to the possible subcategories of comprehension impairment that can be found at an early age. If some very young children do show comprehension deficits without the full syndrome of verbal auditory agnosia, it is essential that their auditory decoding abilities be developed.

The Landau–Kleffner syndrome is less familiar to therapists generally, but there are now some guidelines for intervention emerging as the condition is more effectively recognised. Vance (1991), in a case study of a child with acquired epileptic aphasia (onset at 3;6), describes in detail a structured programme of language re-education and re-emergence. Starting with fundamental bottom-up skills such as auditory detection and discrimination, Vance delineates the slow but effective progress through a predominantly visual approach to language learning, including provision for signing (Paget–Gorman), extensive articulation work and the Colour Coding Scheme. Despite the level of expertise, Vance's charge eventually joined a school with a total-signing environment: a recognition of the poor prognosis in auditory abilities of some of these children.. The need for further research into the intervention practices with such children is proposed by Lees (1993), possibly based, she suggests, on neuropsychological principles. This was attempted by Martin and Reilly (1995). These authors describe, again, a case study of a child with what they term a Central Auditory Processing disorder. (Martin and Reilly propose this is a 'milder' version of Verbal Auditory Agnosia). In contrast to Vance's bottom-up approach, Martin and Reilly aimed for a top-down approach, where little attention was paid to basic auditory skills. There are similarities to other cases in that this child also required, ultimately a visual approach through gesture and the written word. Martin and Reilly's study is an important one because it attempts to apply the framework of cognitive neuropsychology to a developmental disorder, albeit somewhat retrospectively. This is a topic that we will take up again in Chapter 8.

Semantic–pragmatic language disorder

We agree with the position taken by Bishop and Rosenbloom (1987) that we have here a range of conditions rather than one syndrome. This may be briefly exemplified by contrasting the following case with that of the child F given in Chapter 5.

> A was first seen at the age of 4;0 years. He had shown normal developmental milestones following an induced birth at 31 weeks due to maternal hypertension. Forceps were employed and there was a delay in onset of respiration. At the time of his referral, his expressive language was fluent but with some syntactic errors. Some echoic speech was evident. Responses to comprehension items on the RDLS were inconsistent. An overall score of 2;3 years was obtained. He indulged in a considerable amount of monologue during play. Fine motor control was poor. During assessment he showed distractibility and other attention difficulties.
>
> A showed 'unusual and phenomenal skill at reading'. He could read complex instructions at sight (e.g. the psychologist's test sheet) but without understanding. At one point, he scored 170 on the Schonell graded reading test. These attributes place him in the category of hyperlexic children. He was subsequently diagnosed as autistic. However, after 2 years in a special nursery group he was transferred to a mainstream primary class. He continued to show conceptual–semantic problems. Although he had some difficulty in forming relationships with other people he could no longer be considered autistic.

Both A and F showed well-developed syntactic and phonological skills but their expressive language was inappropriate to the situations they were in or to the people they were with. However A had the special feature of his reading skill and showed sufficient signs of autistic behaviour to be so classified for a period of his development. The diagnosis of autism was never considered in F's case.

In discussing semantic–pragmatic disorders, we do not wish to become too involved in the present controversy as to whether or not such behaviour is always associated with autism. We expect to see less extreme views being propagated as more information becomes available. Many speech and language therapists' opposition to the possibility that some of their language-disordered children are autistic is based on faulty understanding of the changing nature of autism. It is not always appreciated that autistic children improve and develop over time. As they do so, different manifestations of their autism become more or less dominant. Autism, like language disorder, is not an absolute state within which no change is to be expected. Children with semantic–pragmatic disorders of language may show autistic features and children who are autistic will have difficulty with semantic–pragmatic aspects of language. We suggest that the decision as to who should work with them be based upon which professional has most to offer the child at any particular period of their development and there is also ample opportunity for joint work between teachers, psychologists and speech and language therapists. Because we are now in a position to define and assess the language disorders that children with autistic features may show, it is logical and humane to develop programmes of language therapy for them.

We would therefore like to make a number of points in relation to intervention for children with semantic–pragmatic disorders. These children typically show a lack of interest in interacting with other people. Some of them are very unresponsive during early childhood and give the impression of general cognitive delay. 'He was difficult to stimulate and difficult to communicate with. He would sit in his pushchair like a little doll paying little attention to activities around him.' Present thinking will therefore encourage the development of interaction between the child and others. Whilst this is extremely important, we believe it should be handled with care. During their early development, the children may need some protection from the battering of an environment, much of which they cannot understand. Continual pressure towards interaction will be fatiguing and could be harmful.

Throughout therapy and education, emphasis should be on the semantic aspect of the condition. These children are unable to appreciate the contextual significance of words. Thus they have comprehension deficits that are testable and functional problems that are continually revealed.

> When he was 6 he started in infant school. The headmistress did not understand his problem. She told him once to pick up litter. He did so but did not put it in the bin. He found it hard to follow even simple instructions and could not follow them through to their logical conclusion. Each day, on the way to school we practised saying 'Please tell me again slowly'. He still makes the same request at 16.

One other brief illustration reminds us of the impossibility of teaching every language nuance. Mother: 'Oh, the alarm's gone off.' Child: 'No, it's gone on'.

Intervention must first attempt to develop simple comprehension through the use of speech in function. Requests for actions rather than for speech should be made. Activities should next be introduced in which the child can use simple speech to direct the adult. Some suggestions may be found in Warner, Byers Brown and McCartney (1984). Throughout the early stages of intervention an attempt to avoid giving ammunition for further semantic–pragmatic manifestations should be made. Thus talking too much and at a level above the child's understanding should be avoided. This will only encourage inattention. Modelling should only be used when the utterance is clearly related to an activity that the child can understand. Otherwise only further stereotyped utterance is being encouraged. Simple labelling should be discouraged. F when shown a picture of a house immediately launched into a catalogue of 'that's a window, that's a door, that's a chimney' etc. without being able to say anything about their function. Word meanings should not be assumed to have been absorbed after one demonstration. They must be continually used and demonstrated in a functional manner employing different situations, rather in the manner described for criterion-referenced assessments in Chapter 6. If the child is able to tolerate, then enjoy interactions, he may be introduced into a small group programme such as that described by Aldred (1983). The functional communicative aspect of language can be reinforced, leaving the therapist or teacher individual time to work on word meanings.

The child must still be encouraged to take an active part and here a metalinguistic approach may be very helpful in reinforcing semantic aspects. For example, he may draw a 'big' man, sitting in the 'big' chair or give Mummy a 'big' kiss. This working and reworking of words in context is one of the most important features of intervention and is one that will continue throughout education, making use of reading and writing as well as speech. It involves teaching the child to 'know' about language. These children have strengths in motor planning and execution and also in some aspects of auditory processing because their speech is clear and intelligible. In order to convert these strengths into assets they need systematic teaching to support their weaknesses at the following levels:

- Conceptual level: intention to speak, appreciation of turn taking, symbol acquisition.
- Abstract level: semantic appreciation, recognition and memory, creation of functional language structures.
- Auditory/receptive level: ability to relate incoming information to meaningful concepts.
- Linguistic level: application of linguistic rules deduced through generalisation.
- Feedback circuits: regulation of behaviour, self-monitoring.

A central constituent of intervention lies, therefore, in the cognitive domain. The semantically- and pragmatically-impaired child presents a complex picture of cognitive deficit. Stimulation of thought processes must proceed concurrently with the teaching of language form and function. Assistance in constructing teaching procedures may therefore be gleaned from texts about children's thought as well as from classic language pathology texts (Wiig and Semel, 1980; Wiig, 1987). Additional information about the approaches to the classroom management of the older children with semantic–pragmatic language disorder is given in Smedley (1989) and Hyde Wright and Cray (1991).

Although it is important not to capitalise and over promote phenomena such as reading without understanding (barking at print), it is very important to cultivate genuine talents.

> At the age of 8 he began recorder lessons. He could not read music but enjoyed making a noise and 'played' in assembly with the group. I taught him to mime. He just had to watch the other children and follow their lead.
> Then, at 9 years he began flute lessons with an old student friend who knew about his problems. As there were only two flautists in the junior school he became a 'star', in his own eyes anyway. Self-esteem causes a person to grow and his natural talent began to show. His flute became his means of communicating his feelings and he plays with great sensitivity.

Today this boy (aged 16) is a member of his local youth orchestra and choir. He plays the piano and the piccolo in addition to the flute. He has passed seven subjects in his General Certificate of Education examinations and is to take music and another subject at 'A' level. His written language is still 'chatty' and unstructured, but he is very strongly motivated to improve. He had a very severe semantic–pragmatic problem in childhood and his improvement is due to a combination of inspired and loving home support and strong self-motivation. His parents were told when he was 2 years of age that he was severely subnormal 'with no meaningful future'.

Developmental verbal dyspraxia

Although the most salient presenting feature in verbal dyspraxia may be the articulatory/phonological deficit, we have found from clinical experience that this is not a fruitful level at which to begin a programme of intervention. Perhaps reasons for this will become clear when the features that characterise developmental dyspraxic disorders are considered. The description given in Chapter 5 included two major points, the first being that this is not a unitary disorder but that rather in the same way that the semantic–pragmatic disorder occurs on a continuum of severity so it is the case with DVD (Crary, 1984, 1993). Some types of the disorder appear to derive from higher-order linguistic processing (i.e.

they are more 'aphasic' in nature) and others resemble errors in motor processing (i.e. they are more 'dysarthric'). It is of interest to note that Tempest and Parkinson (1993) are of the opinion that DVD is due to problems of the storage of phonological form in memory (thus raising interesting parallels with other more 'linguistic' types of SLI), rather than a condition restricted to phonological output processing or motoric process constraints. The second point made in the description was that because of incomplete language development in children the disorder is more likely to manifest itself as being predominantly linguistically determined (a fact which may account for Tempest and Parkinson's hypothesis).

There are two broadly connected areas on which intervention must be focused. These are:

- Non-segmental aspects.
- Segmental aspects.

We consider it essential to begin with the first. Developmentally this seems to make sense, for non-segmental aspects of language are both understood and produced before segmental forms. Furthermore, as was described in Chapter 4, linguistic processing of prosodic features probably take place well upstream in the production chain. Prosodic disorders are therefore seen as an intrinsic part of DVD and not as overlaid features resulting from a primary motor deficit. Byers Brown and Lewis (1984) and Byers Brown (1988) have drawn attention to a group of children who showed preference for vowel sequences /uh uh uh/ which they used referentially and with variation in volume. It was suggested that this was a communicative strategy adopted by the children who had not yet developed adequate motor schemata. In planning remediation one needs to consider the components of prosody, the tone-group, tone and tonicity. Additionally stress, rhythm and pause are important. Twelve out of the 13 children in the Edwards' pilot study showed difficulties in signalling change in stress, rhythm and intonation. Their response in assessment tasks where a change of stress indicated a change of meaning tended towards syllabic type speech with equal and even stress.

It is probably best to begin with a general rhythmic programme by making the child aware of the properties of prosody. This can be undertaken by the use of rhymes and jingles. Not only is it necessary to aim for rhythmic production, but the appreciation of changes in pitch direction and in stress patterns is also very important. The child needs to listen to demonstrations of change and to be able to identify their nature. Because many of these children have an associated motor problem (clumsiness) it may be fruitful to gradually introduce a rhythmic motor activity concomitantly with the language work. Tapping movements that accompany speech are sometimes useful, but this should be self-generated and not imposed by an outside source like a metronome. It is stressed that there is not a cause–effect relationship between movement difficulties and DVD. Motor programmes for each are separately determined.

Visual cues may be very helpful. For older children, writing out phrases with indication of stress and pitch change is one way of doing this. For younger children, Kellett has developed a colour scheme using blocks; for example the change in pitch direction is demonstrated by placing the nuclear stress block at a higher level in a row representing the utterance (Kellett, Lee and Mobley, 1984). Visispeech also offers both a model and feedback. Mirror work is sometimes suggested, but our own experience of this has been very unsatisfactory. In one case it produced such frustration in a child that he broke down completely and spat at his own image.

Segmental speech problems require an approach different from that which might be adopted for an articulatory disorder. The overall emphasis is on sequence rather than on individual sounds. DVD is characterised by sequential errors that may be anticipatory, perseverative or metathetic. There is therefore little point in concentrating on sound production for it is not a case of inability to produce, but rather one where the ordering of sounds constitutes the main problem. If there is a good foundation of work on establishing normal prosodic patterns, there will already be a framework into which sequences can be slotted. Rosenbek (1974) advocates reduplicating syllable sequences using CV combinations that the child already finds relatively easy to produce. The emphasis is on slowness, and on self-monitoring. He suggests a mix of nonsense sounds and real words, the former being favoured at first because they obviate the recurrence of previous learning errors. Babbling exercises as such are not thought to be useful, for in fact they only succeed in taking the child back to a much earlier stage of development and the relationship of babbling to subsequent language is in any case not a straightforward one.

Also we do not see much value in exercises of articulatory organs. In the first place they serve no functional neurophysiological purpose in relation to speech and, secondly, it is generally agreed that the best way to improve speech is by speaking.

Reference has already been made to concomitant syntactic disorders. The work of Panagos, Quine and Klich (1979) has shown the close interrelationship which exists on a two-way basis between phonological and syntactic complexity. The explanation of reduced syntax through an economy of effort strategy really is untenable. It should therefore be borne in mind that there is a need to balance the two aspects, i.e. when working at phonological level to resort to uncomplicated syntactic forms and vice versa. Auditory discrimination work per se has yielded disappointing results (Yoss and Darley, 1974b).

Associated problems

Reading and writing problems of a nature somewhat similar to those of speech frequently occur. This is hardly surprising for, covertly, spoken and written language may share a common processing system. Stackhouse (1982, 1985) has carried out a series of studies examining the nature of reading and spelling deficits in dyspraxic children. She found the errors to be qualitatively different from those attributable to a disorder that was predominantly phonetic in nature. Commenting on the diversity and idiosyncrasy of the errors she considers that this may be an indication of different subgroups of the disorder.

The close link between the disorder of spoken and written language obviously calls for very close cooperative work between teachers and therapists so that a common strategy may be determined. Failure to do this could result in even greater confusion for a child who may already be very frustrated. Where the disorder is very severe, placement in a language unit is highly desirable. In this way joint work can be carried out more satisfactorily. There is also a better opportunity to pace the amount of work. Over-intensity of input can be deleterious in that it may exacerbate perseverative tendencies. Tempest and Parkinson (1993) advocated a team approach to phonological therapy and reading development with a case of severe dyspraxia. They found the blending of the visual written form and articulation training techniques, along with the teaching of phonological awareness to be successful.

Phonologic–syntactic language disorder

It has been pointed out several times that this is the largest of the clinical subgroups of language disorder. It is the one that is most likely to constitute the bulk of the language unit population. However, we must be aware of circular arguments. Although it qualifies for that position by numerical representation, it also qualifies by reason of suitability. The consensus of opinion seems to be that these children may safely be admitted to units or looked after in the mainstream school because their comprehension is sufficiently developed to allow them to understand what is going on. They do not need the protection of a special school unless their difficulties are extremely severe and/or compounded by other factors.

Children with phonological–syntactic problems may first present with delayed speech. If they are still very young, prophylactic measures may be instituted (see Chapter 3). It is desirable that the therapist study the child and monitor his or her progress over a period of time in order to obtain some idea of their rate of growth. Certain principles of phonology, syntax and semantics may be absorbed and acted upon during these early years. Attention may be controlled and fostered on the lines described by Cooper, Moodley and Reynell (1978). It was suggested (Byers Brown, 1971) that during this period it might be possible to observe whether the child was developing a linguistic system in a fragmented manner, or whether it was cohesive but constrained. Intervention will therefore be carried out to help the child either to organise his system or to expand it.

During the preschool years changes may occur in either direction. For example, attention may improve or attention difficulties may remain and show increased relationship to general cognitive impairment. Motor skills may improve or there may be a gradual revelation of subtle coordination difficulties. There may be improvement in ability to generate words in order, but continued difficulty in phonological planning leading to unintelligibility. We have already drawn attention to the finding by Bishop and Edmundson (1987b) that the more areas involved the poorer the prognosis. Any or all of the following areas of deficit may be found. At linguistic level: phonological representation, storage and retrieval; creation of planning frame; insertion of phonological forms into planning frame; generation and retrieval of specific linguistic forms; application of phonetic rules. At motor level: retrieval of appropriate motor schemata; generation of neuromuscular programme; articulatory presentation. Feedback circuits: feedforward of auditory and motor information to allow planning; feedback via proprioception.

The following case history indicates how some of the impairments at different levels become apparent during development.

I was referred at 2;0 years because of the absence of words. Auditory acuity and middle ear function were normal and there was no delay in any other parameters of development. Speech sound behaviour consisted of jargon, vowels with intonation and vocalisations. This would be considered normal for a child of around 12 months. A programme of language stimulation and parent guidance (in which both parents took part) was instituted. During the next 18 months I suffered several episodes of otitis media raising the question as to whether or not this could have been a factor contributing to his speech delay. Although his hearing was normal when tested there is no guarantee that this was always the case. However, as his parents were alert to the possibility of fluctuating hearing loss and brought him regularly for assessment, it was considered an unlikely contributor to language delay.

At 3;8 I showed a language comprehension age of 3;5 and an expressive age of 2;4 years. The overall pattern was one of slow growth. However, he had made expressive gains of about 16 months in a 20-month period. In order to determine whether this was a resolving delay or a disorder the pattern of language development must be looked at. The following characteristics were noted: high proportion of nouns in relation to other words, telegraphic utterances, failure to observe word boundaries, late emergence of phonological system, continuing use of gesture. Intervention accordingly shifted to a solid programme of language building, learning new words, memorising rhymes and word games, the child giving word directives and listening to stories read by the mother or therapist in order to retell them. I was able to manage in normal primary school with therapy support and appeared to be functioning normally when he entered junior school. No educational difficulties were reported. It seems likely that I's difficulties were at the linguistic level, particularly affecting planning. This appeared to be strengthened by the measures taken. I never showed pragmatic difficulties. His good cognitive ability was demonstrated in his progress and was always apparent to his parents.

Early therapy should provide the young language-delayed child with more information or help him to organise the information he possesses. It attempts to guide him through the stages of progressive differentiation and make the right choices at the right time. The therapist must therefore be aware of the features that she is attempting to control or modify. What are the language units that the child is producing and that he appears able to handle? What units does he need to round out his system? Will he be able to deduce rules for himself if stimulated by simple speech that is interesting to him and that contains considerable repetition and redundancy? Or, does he need to be taught a few discriminations in a direct manner? Such information can well be learned through interacting with the child in a simple natural manner that will allow him to converse. This will show how much he is able to follow the lead of an adult speaker, to pattern his speech upon that of the therapist and to experiment with speech and language forms.

Theoretical advances in the field of grammatical language impairment are impacting on the direction of the development of intervention strategies. Van der Lely produces some 'tentative' indications for therapy based on her work with children who have persistent problems in the processing of grammatical information, and who are impaired in their ability to accrue information about the syntactic constituents of utterances. Given that the children Van der Lely (1993) tested had difficulty in this area, she suggests the use of strategies to introduce words (in this case, verbs) in situations where their semantic properties can be learnt, and to then present these same verbs to the child in many different sentence frames. In this way, the child has the task of decoding simplified for him or her. The semantic information is made explicit, so that the child can focus on the syntactic task.

Recent research (Bishop, 1983, 1987b; Van der Lely and Dewart, 1986; Adams, 1990) has now revealed that children with such disorders may be suffering from subtle deficits of comprehension that only become apparent as the language to which they are exposed becomes more complex (see also the discussion of R as cited in Chapter 5). This may be checked by steady reappraisal and reassessment of the child's functional levels. However, although these children may have passed earlier assessment tests at appropriate levels, functional comprehension difficulty is observed frequently by the therapist. As one becomes familiar with the child's personality and overall behaviour, one develops greater sensitivity to even slight changes. A delay in response or momentary confusion will signal lack of comprehension and this may be tackled immediately. If a parent is present (and in the case of individual therapy this is extremely likely), advice may be given as to how to deal with such signs when they are observed at home.

Gibson and Ingram (1983), in a diary account of the development of comprehension and production in a language-delayed child over a period of 17 months, provide valuable information about changes that took place. Progress was characterised by a series of spurts that coincided with changes in developmental milestones. The authors suggest that this might be one way in which clinicians can capitalise on normal growth to stimulate progress in language.

Within the considerable span of this clinical subtype there can be a wide range of symptoms and signs and, of course, severity. Children who are identified at the stage of language delay may be well documented by the time they reach 5;0 years of age. The rate of their progress, its even or uneven nature and the factors that appear to influence it, may be helpfully described. It should be becoming apparent whether the child is going to manage within the normal school or whether they will need provision in a unit or in a special school. Concurrent with this will be the decision to embark on a teaching programme based upon the child's individual language profile. The popularity of the Derbyshire Language Scheme testifies to the need that units have to make use of some developed scheme. Other children may be considered suitable candidates for the highly structured methods advised by Hutt (1986) and propagated through ICAN. Such decisions are made in accordance with the avowed policy of unit or school as well as in the interests of individual children. The present weight of evidence seems to show that it is unwise to embark on a structured scheme before the child has been observed and worked with over a period of time and during the early developmental period. If they are a late referral or a very severe case, they may merit special consideration. Harris's (1984) valuable discussion is likely to remain particularly pertinent to all questions of this kind.

Lexical–syntactic language disorder deficit

German (1985, 1987, 1992) has studied this deficit extensively as have also Wiig and Semel (1984) and Wiig and Becker-Caplan (1984). It is a disorder that may not readily be apparent. The child may be thought of as being quiet and non-communicative because of the sparseness of spoken language. In contrast to the quiet children there are those who appear to be almost garrulous with a near incessant flow of talk. Both types require careful investigation so that appropriate remediation can be undertaken.

In the first instance a combination of formal testing (e.g. The Test of Word Finding, German, 1989) and analysis of a spontaneous sample of speech may help to identify certain classes of words that present difficulties of retrieval for the child. In the second case, it is likely that closer investigation of spontaneous speech will reveal a fair amount of emptiness. This needs to be viewed very carefully for we are all prone to use filler pauses and it was pointed out in Chapter 4 that these 'non-fluencies' probably signify stretches of active planning of speech. But abnormality is indicated by the amount of meaningless insertions that usually precede content words. (Crystal (1981) incidentally calls into question definitions of and distinctions between content and function words.) Typical of this emptiness is 'Well.... Well we went to this kind of er place and then we put on these things and we sort of we played this game' (this represents an account of going to another school to play football). Speech is characterised by revision, by repair and by obvious searches for the word. Interestingly the same phenomenon is apparent in the speech of many normal elderly people, although here it is concentrated more specifically on names. We have made reference to syntagmatic and paradigmatic associations that occur in a developmental sequence. This factor needs to be borne in mind in planning remedial work as do other categorisations.

The aims of remedial work are to enlarge the child's 'internal dictionary' and to build up associative networks that facilitate access to vocabulary. Direct and fairly structured intervention may focus on the characteristics of words, both 'semantic' and 'phonological'. The aim is to enrich the child's knowledge of the properties of the referent, by contrasting the conceptual information attached to it with related items. It has also been proposed that phonological enrichment is important (McGregor and Leonard, 1995). So the child would need to learn about the phonological structure of the word and be able to participate in activities with a set of phonologically-related words. The other crucial dichotomy that underpins the framework of intervention with these children is the 'storage vs retrieval' debate referred to in Chapter 5 (p. 131). Intervention studies in this area have suffered from methodological problems, but there is now increasingly satisfactory evidence to support the notion that both elaboration and retrieval activities combined together in one remedial programme is the optimal and effective treatment method (Hyde Wright, 1993; McGregor and Leonard, 1995). As further information becomes available regarding the nature of these children's difficulties, we should be in a position to more accurately direct intervention based on developmental psycholinguistic principles. The relationship of word-finding to reading and spelling deficits is also now emerging (Stackhouse, 1993), and it is likely that the two skills are linked at some underlying level of processing. Gathercole (1994) proposes that word-learning deficits may be based on problems of phonological short-term memory, and that this may be the fundamental impairment that leads to broader language learning problems. She advocates rehearsal training and continued and repetitive practice at retrieval to ameliorate the memory problems. These methods have yet to be tested out empirically. A recurring theme is that it is important that therapy for word-finding problems should address the central vocabulary deficit and that the net should not be cast too widely. 'Word finding interventions should be sufficiently focused to provide some critical experiences' (McGregor and Leonard, 1995, pp. 95–96).

It would be unwise to assume that direct intervention strategies will be all that is required in the approach to the management of word-finding difficulties. These deficits have the reputation of being some of the most persistent language problems. In particular, it is not uncommon to record cases that have word-finding deficits as the sole residual impairment after an earlier more global deficit. If one expects as part of the prognosis that there will be residual difficulties, then there is a need to maximise the compensatory strategies that can be made available to the child. German (1992) makes some suggestions in this area. As a complement to the vocabulary and retrieval practice in therapy, she outlines the need for the child/student to adopt strategies to cue themselves into words as they have been taught in remedial sessions. But there is also a crucial requirement for the educational environment to be modified to help the child. Both German (1992) and McGregor and Leonard (1995) emphasise that the teacher and speech and language therapist must work together to 'restructure the environment' (German, p. 48), for instance by allowing extra time to answer questions. (See McGregor and Leonard (1995) for the most comprehensive review of this area.)

Phonological disorder

It is not proposed to describe intervention here, for the emphasis throughout the description of language disorders has focused on syndromes. Moreover, it has been shown that in the majority of cases, phonological disorders occur in conjunction with deficits at other levels. That is not to say that they do not merit specialised intervention; on the contrary the amount of detail required in analysis and planning of treatment precludes a description in this text.

This decade has seen a huge surge of interest in one specific technique for the remediation of phonological impairment (in the UK, at least) and that is the Metaphon technique (Howell and Dean, 1994). Having designed this metalinguistic assessment and remedial procedure, Howell and Dean describe its extensive use in research and clinic work. Using natural process analysis they base their work on Piagetian constructs and on increasing the child's metalinguistic awareness of the sound system. It is mainly in the course of intervention that the metalinguistic strategies are encouraged and production work is minimised until later stages. Metaphon encourages the child to take an active part in therapy by learning about the properties of sounds. This process of learning is claimed to be the means by which children can change the way in which they process sounds and sound contrasts, especially from an output point of view. There is, however, continuing debate regarding the supposed novelty of such techniques (see Dean et al., 1995 and Grundy, 1995b). Grundy, quite rightly, points out that this is not a metalinguistic, but a metaphonetic technique. Overall, Van Kleek (1981) considers that the functions of metalinguistic skills have considerable value in clinical application. However, Howard and Hesketh (1993), debate the structure of the Metaphon programme, and question the necessity of carrying out all of the different stages in the order specified, concluding that 'for children who are consistently unable to make metalinguistic judgements it may be that a different approach to phonological remediation may be preferable' (p. 7). There was phonological therapy before Metaphon, of course, and in fact the programme itself is a collection of various techniques that have been in common usage for many years, with specific and very innovative modifications to appeal to the young child. Space does not permit a full review of alternative sources of guidance for phonological therapy. The reader is directed to Stackhouse (1984), Weiss, Gordon and Lillywhite (1987), Creaghead, Newman and Secord (1989), Dodd (1995) for further reading.

Throughout this chapter, we have considered types of intervention that the speech and language therapist may utilise; in other words, we have focused on methodological aspects, the speech and language therapy process. An equally important feature that has a significant contribution to make to the success of the therapeutic endeavour is the dyadic relationship between child and therapist. The focus on interactive aspects of intervention is growing (e.g. Letts, 1985). Ripich and Panagos (1985), Panagos, Bobkoff and Scott (1986), and Panagos et al., (1988) have employed discourse theory to analyse clinical procedures. This they have applied to both verbal and non-verbal interaction. The clinical session is divided into lesson, task and remedial sequence. Under the first heading is included the opening phase when greetings are exchanged, questions are asked about progress etc. The work phase concentrates on the task in hand for the current session and the closing phase includes reminders, future plans and farewell greetings. The task phase begins with instructions and illustrations, then moves on to the actual procedures and is finalised by discussion of the next steps to be taken in the process of therapy. The remedial sequence relates to actual therapeutic techniques, the request for a particular response and the evaluation of that response. For many clinicians, this is a familiar routine that is adopted subconsciously. Nevertheless an analysis of interactive elements may be helpful in revealing reasons for specific failures and successes in therapy.

Chapter 8
Reflections and future developments

Summary

This chapter considers some of the issues that present challenges to therapists and researchers for the immediate future. The issue of taxonomy is addressed, in addition to a discussion of some of the professional challenges of working with children with developmental language disorders into the next millennium.

Taxonomy and definitions

One intention of this final chapter was to consider whether a firm taxonomy of developmental language disorder is a realistic possibility. The progression of our ideas with the growth of the writing leads us to think that this is not the most fruitful way at the present time towards furthering knowledge. Description of early language development, prophylactic measures, the gradual shading of immature language into full blown disorders all serve to confirm the notion of language and language disorder being on a continuum ranging from normality through to deviance. Within the category of deviance too we have not found it helpful to recognise discrete entities for they share commonalities. Language as one of the most complex aspects of human behaviour does not readily lend itself to strict taxonomy. It seems therefore that labels will always have to be accompanied by description and by explanation if remediation is to meet with success. One of the chief values of a classification system is that, having identified a particular type of disorder, we should then be in a strong position to recommend the most suitable type of intervention. We have considered this in the light of available resources at the present time.

As our ability to identify particular types of language disorder grows, we may hope to seek out the specific components of these disorders within other populations of handicapped children. In this text, the emphasis has been on those children for whom language disorder is the essential handicap. We know that it may also occur in children who are intellectually-impaired, hearing-impaired or who have cerebral palsies. Such children will need a combination of intervention approaches to enable them to cope with their combined handicaps. As we gain more assurance in the areas of intervention for language disorder, we must ensure that the needs of multiply-handicapped children are met.

The relationship of language impairment to other conditions is likely to remain a focus of keen interest and research for many years. This is not merely an academic debate. The outcome of it will have significant implications for the targeting of scarce resources of speech and language intervention. The task is to examine the relationship between three categories of language impairment, (which may appear to have validity on paper at present, in practice and in the future so that we may be able to overcome superficial demarcations and to define interrelations more specifically. These may be described as:

- specific: where the language impairment stands alone in the absence of an explanatory factor;
- general: where the language impairment is associated with another condition or a developmental delay;
- pervasive: where the language impairment is associated with social and cognitive developmental deficits (see Chapter 5).

Specific developmental language impairment is increasingly something of an endangered species. A synthesis of research findings, case studies, as well as increased professional awareness of the learning-disabled populations and academic debate, is gradually steering a course away from a fixed notion of a pure entity of language disorder. Here, a principle focus of discussion has been the use of mental age criteria as a means of identifying the child with specific language impairment (Lahey, 1990). The assumption that a verbal/non-verbal IQ discrepancy can adequately identify the child with a specific language impairment has been called into question. Lahey argues that the definition and description of 'intelligence' into neat categories of ability may be erroneous. 'If autonomy exists among domains of intelligence, is there any value in identifying a problem by comparing one domain with another?' (Lahey, 1990, p. 616). This contention has been lent material support by the research of Cole and his colleagues, (Cole, Dale and Mills, 1990; Cole et al., 1995).

Cole et al. (1995) examined the stability of diagnosis of children categorised as either specific language impairment (IQ in normal range) or developmental lag language impaired (IQ and language performance both significantly behind chronological age), by two methods: exclusionary criteria or IQ discrepancy (Cole et al. refer to the second method as 'cognitive referencing'). By following up their subjects over time they were able to map out the changes in language and cognitive performance that occurred in both groups. The notable result of their studies is that individual children could be seen to be crossing the borders from specific language impairment to developmental lag language impairment and vice versa over time. Cole et al. conclude that 'the results of this study lead us to question the usefulness of the classification of SLI because of the low stability for the classification using either definition' (Cole et al., 1995, p. 115). It clearly makes little clinical common sense that children might exist in one group at one time and another a year later. Speech and language therapists and specialist teachers are well aware of the constellation of learning difficulties and subtle cognitive and motor deficits that accompany the diagnosis of specific language impairment. It may therefore be an apposite time to reflect of the future use of such terminology and the alternative diagnostic procedures that might need to be implemented.

It is imperative that more attention in terms of empirical research and intervention priorities be directed at the language-impaired child with additional learning difficulties. Research is beginning to show that this group may be at greater risk for long-term social and academic deficits than more able language-impaired children. The inference from Stothard et al.'s (1996) follow-up of children who received speech and language therapy as preschoolers, is that less able children may require more intensive and pro-active intervention and support in the early years. An examination of the targeting of resources to children with language impairment, perhaps placed in a special needs or moderate learning difficulties environment would be timely.

Intervention methods and research

Changing beliefs about definitions of language impairment lends support to an urgent requirement for more experimentation in order that we understand more fully the group of conditions we are calling developmental language disorders. But as a clinical profession there is also an overriding need for sound intervention studies, either large or small scale, so that we can more accurately pinpoint which types of intervention are most effective with particular groups. New methods of intervention are worth reporting and sharing with fellow professionals. The situation is perhaps better now than some years ago, and there is a large number of single case studies available for the clinician to consult. But there is still some reluctance to share ideas and information in a written form. From small-scale pilot projects to large, group studies of efficacy, there should be sharing and dissemination of ideas about therapy in order to stimulate greater confidence in the profession about the methods of intervention used with these children.

Intervention research has other benefits than those of pure clinical replication. By studying the effects of manipulation of the environment on the process of language learning, and by observing the changes with instruction in a disordered mechanism, we might hope to gain valuable insight in to the nature of language and language acquisition itself. Intervention research might be, as Ellis Weismer (1991) puts it, 'the ultimate challenge in terms of testing our theoretical constructs of language learning and the nature of language disorders'. The reality of the situation is that intervention research is unattractive to academics, who are relatively removed from daily clinical contact, because of the complexities, expense and necessary 'messiness' of the methodologies involved. One of the inherent features of intervention research is that lengthy periods of time will have to be spent with the subjects. Clinicians are in an ideal position to carry out such research, but may lack the funding, the time or the confidence. The way out of this dilemma is to provide support for the clinicians to carry out research and for funding bodies to prioritise intervention research. Despite the drawbacks of the economics of such enterprise, the far-reaching consequences of a failure to address these issues will be a persistence of ignorance about the effectiveness of therapeutic intervention.

Effectiveness of therapy

Accountability, clinical audit, quality assurance–these are some of the buzz terms of the 1990s for health service professionals. The notion of reflection on quality and models of delivery of service for the language-impaired as part of an overall provision of care is a relatively recent one–at least in such explicit terms. If we are to function in an environment of introspection and self-examination, it is even more necessary than ever that we have accurate data about intervention techniques and the delivery of skilled intervention and long-term educational provision for children with developmental language disorders. In the days of 'evidence-based medicine' it is imperative that issues of effectiveness are investigated by those who have a broad base of understanding of the condition and the individualisation of issues, rather than by economists who focus on gross outcome measures.

The consensus of opinion in the literature is that therapy for children with language impairments is effective (Nye, Foster and Seaman, 1987; Ellis Weismer, 1991; Enderby and Emerson, 1995). Kluppel (1991) justifies her claim that 'there are no unresolvable problems facing investigators interested in the efficacy of intervention applied to children with language disorders', by systematically examining the problems and providing realistic solutions to them. Enderby and Emerson call for the investigation of many more regimes of therapy and make a start by initiating a large scale study of early intervention with language-delayed children (Glogowska, 1996); utilising a rarely used method, (in speech-language therapy at least), randomised controlled trialling.

For an intervention regime to be considered effective it should have a number of qualities that extend far beyond simply doing somebody some good. The following considerations for evaluation might be made:

- It should be effective–the intervention should result in a change in behaviour in the desired direction over and above what might be expected by maturation.
- It should be replicable–not only in terms of adequate description of techniques, but also the effects should not depend on the 'super-clinician effect', i.e. the possibility that an exceptional clinician might have produced the results from sheer personality and force of character.
- It should be realistic in economic terms. Ellis Weismer refers to the dilemma of researching intervention regimes where the investigator adopts the ideal strategy of intervention, achieves remarkable results in terms of effectiveness, but where the project has little generalisation value because the proposed model implies an unachievable increase in resources. Intervention effectiveness research should strive to reflect the realities of economic constraint as far as possible.
- It should be targeted at the right population. Of all the current dilemmas in evidence-based intervention this is perhaps the most difficult one to address. How can we know which intervention strategies will be of maximum effectiveness for a particular group of children at a given stage of development? 'As a profession we often do not know which children are in most need of that intervention and are unlikely to improve if therapy is not available' (Glogowska, 1996).

In the new world of the NHS, with purchasing agreements and efficiency savings, it is now the case that British speech and language therapists are facing much the same pressures to produce evidence of treatment efficacy that our counterparts in America have had for some time. At the same time the recognition of poor communication as having a profound affect on life outcomes in so many ways has extended the remit of therapists to include a much wider range of age and disability. A satisfactory way to deal with these pressures has yet to be achieved in the working lives of many therapists.

The theoretical underpinning of intervention

Perhaps the greatest challenge for the speech and language therapist working with children with developmental language disorders is the immense diversity and complexity of the theoretical background. Theories in this discipline, however, do not generally support the process of intervention in the way that they do with other major areas of speech-language pathology. It is notable that one can identify easily specific techniques and methods to be used with, say, adults who stutter, and many of these will be based on an identifiable theory of the cause of stuttering. Of course there is no proven theory of stuttering, but this has not stood in the way of the evolution of disparate methods for the treatment of advanced dysfluency. This begs the question as to why there has been a relative lack of congruence between theory of language impairment in children and models of intervention. This inconstant position has probably arisen for several reasons:

- the diversity and individuality of the children affected and the need to tailor intervention closely to their particular needs and interests;
- the changing nature of the language achievements and profiles of these children over time;
- the requirement to integrate language learning work with educational goals;
- the amount of knowledge required of the therapist, in terms of normal language development from early levels of vocabulary and syntactic development, up to the higher levels of semantic and pragmatic ability;
- the resultant amount of knowledge required to resource and support this diverse and complex set of disorders.

Future directions in intervention: top-down and bottom-up approaches

The absence of explanatory theories in the intervention process has not precluded an accumulation of models of support of that process. The advent of linguistics as a framework for understanding developmental language disorders provided the profession with a way to look at the parts, but left the 'whole picture' somewhat out in the cold. It may have provided us with sophisticated analytical tools leading to a high level of knowledge about the profile of the disorder, but there are no corresponding intervention methods dictated as a direct result. A linguistic approach allows the weaknesses and strengths to be mapped out, or a particular language structure to be pinpointed as an intervention goal. The method of achieving that goal is not provided, and it is up to the clinician to devise a way to plug the gaps in language development. Moreover, because of the lack of an explanatory theory, there is the impression that one is treating the symptoms rather than the cause. Van Der Lely (1993) attempted to redress the balance by directly relating research findings about grammatical impairments in children to intervention, and suggested ways in which they might be taught about the syntactic and semantic properties of verbs.

There is an impression that the limitations of the linguistic approach have been keenly felt and this is recognised in the advent of methods that have attempted to redress the balance.

Top-down approaches

One of the substantial changes in emphasis in models of intervention over the last decade has been the advent of a collection of approaches that might be loosely grouped together as a 'pragmatic method', where the 'method' of intervention is dictated by the functional use of the target behaviour. So natural situations will be used to stimulate and model appropriate language behaviours, rather than teaching language out of context. This corresponds to Fey's hybrid or child-oriented approaches (Fey, Catts and Larrivee, 1995).

An example of such an approach is the Whole Language philosophy, which has gained considerable ground in the US and elsewhere, but which currently is little used in the UK. The underlying rationale of this philosophy, which incorporates a set of diverse approaches, is related to studies of normal language development which advocate that language develops in a whole-to-part fashion (as opposed to the part-to-whole pattern advocated in a bottom-up approach). A critical variable in the process of language learning is seen to be the context in which the language learning takes place. As context is considered to be of crucial importance, it follows that language acquisition will be facilitated by an approach that preserves the natural environment of learning. Consequently 'the wholeness of language is violated by teaching practices in which function, content and form are separated from one another' (Norris and Hoffman, 1993). Gillam, McFadden and Van Kleeck (1995) describe the process of Whole Language therapy as being one in which the child is actively engaged in using language, in listening to stories and talking about them. The Whole Language philosophy has as an integral part the notion that spoken and written language develop hand in hand, and hence probably is more applicable to the older child. But the underlying beliefs substantiate principles that have much to contribute to the intervention debate and that are diametrically opposed to what goes on in some speech and language therapy sessions currently.

Such approaches do not advocate that we abandon linguistic analysis as a tool, or that we should just sit and chat to children with SLI. Rather they assume a confident level of familiarity with the normal progression of language development that can be flexibly and imaginatively integrated into fluid activities. One might associate this set of techniques with a top-down approach to language learning, and it is possible that speech and language therapists are perhaps not so well prepared to deal with these sorts of approaches in their training as they are with the very bottom-up approaches to language therapy, and that to participate in this top-down type of intervention demands considerably more clinical flair and flexibility than bottom-up approaches.

Bottom-up approaches

Many programmes of language intervention might be considered as bottom-up approaches, with their emphasis on building up the units of language systematically. One of the most recent examples of such an approach in that derived from the cognitive neuropsychology processing model. Cognitive neuropsychology as a modern discipline is relatively new in terms of widespread clinical application to language disorders. Cognitive neuropsychologists are interested in how the brain manages to perform complex cognitive operations. Applied to language, one of the original aims of the cognitive neuropsychological school was to attempt to explain the normal processes underlying language function by studying those with brain injuries (Ellis and Young, 1988). Cognitive neuropsychology derives its evidence for the organisation of these complex processes by studying the associations and disassociations of certain processing tasks carried out by the human brain. It relies on the hypothesis that the cognitive system is organised into discrete modules that act independently yet synergistically to perform the complicated and swift task of processing language, both in input and output modes. In acquired language disorder (as a result of cerebral trauma) one ormore of these modules involved in the processing of language becomes incapacitated, and by studying the abilities of certain patients with different lesions, researchers claim to have gathered evidence for the existence and relative independence of some modules, though evidence for the connections between modules has been more difficult to accumulate. The evidence has been assembled into a substantial body of literature, which it would be impossible to review here. The reader is referred to texts by Coltheart, Job and Sartori (1987), Ellis and Young (1988) and Berndt and Mitchum (1995) for further background reading. Speech and language therapists have employed a diagrammatic model of language processing derived from clinical case studies and studies of normal subjects' language processing abilities, in order to guide intervention strategies, in both the fields of acquired and developmental language impairments.

It is notable that some of the pioneering studies in the study of cognitive neuropsychology (e.g. Marshall and Newcombe, 1973), were concerned with the breakdown of the reading and writing systems rather than with spoken language processing. This is reflected in the developmental field where the application of cognitive neuropsychological models are much further advanced in the study of developmental dyslexia (Snowling, 1987), than developmental language disorders. However, although in its infancy, the application of principles of cognitive neuropsychology to the study of developmental language disorders has aroused considerable excitement and enthusiasm within the clinical profession. This may partly be because of the dearth of any other understandable model of language processing on which to formulate hypotheses about the location of the deficit in the language-impaired child, and even less on which to build an appropriate intervention regime. These are both potent reasons for its further examination as a substantial method to add to the therapeutic approaches employed with language-impaired children.

The principle research methodology for cognitive neuropsychologists has been the single case study. Recently a number of developmental cognitive neuropsychological case studies have been presented, and these have been greeted as a welcome extension of debate in an under-researched field. Bryan and Howard (1992) and Stackhouse (1993) have shed light on some of the possible underlying phonological processing deficits in severe overt phonological disorders. Chiat and Hunt (1993) in another case study, show the developmental cognitive neuropsychological approach at its best in the analysis of word-finding deficits and their relationship to underlying phonological processing in a 6-year-old child. There is considerable potential for the developmental cognitive neuropsychological model to enhance our knowledge with respect to phonological and lexical processing in particular (see also the discussion relating to Stackhouse and Wells' work in Chapter 4). Case studies are becoming increasingly sophisticated; for instance, the inclusion of control data is a welcome development (Bryan and North, 1994). The careful extension of the model to children with established language disorders will benefit from cautious and self-critical investigations. Martin and Reilly (1995) employed a developmental cognitive neuropsychological approach to the analysis of a child with a 'global' language deficit, who had very limited comprehension and expression, and was suspected of having auditory processing deficits. The application of the developmental cognitive neuropsychological model to a child with so little in the way of developed language (and the extension to the gestural system of the child) is perhaps less successful. One of the tests of a new model's usefulness would be the extent to which it adds to current thinking or replaces old strategies of intervention. Clearly with very young children who have barely begun to process language the model has limitations.

Developmental cognitive neuropsychology as applied to speech and language disorders has evolved largely from practitioners' use of principles that colleagues have used with adult aphasic clients. This is a clear indication that clinicians desire a strong model on which to base their therapy, and the limitations of previous models, e.g. the linguistic one, in the context of clinical practice. Clinicians are in firm agreement that the hours spent analysing samples to construct an intervention strategy cannot be justified when pressures are continually applied to increase the numbers of children seen. The advantages of the developmental cognitive neuropsychological approach are threefold: firstly it makes clinical common sense for many patients, and clinicians can see for themselves the revelation of processing deficits unmasked. Secondly it has the attraction of clear theoretical underpinnings, and lastly it is relatively quick to assess and design a treatment programme within the model.

The perilous procedure of attempting to draw parallels between language in breakdown and language in acquisition, however, is now well understood. Cognitive neuropsychology as applied to acquired disorders has been a contentious though productive area of research and debate, and there is no reason to suppose that the study of developmental cognitive neuropsychology will differ. One might ask whether it is wise to acquiesce to the widespread adoption of an unproved theoretical framework as a basis for intervention with many children. We know little about the proposed 'modules' in processing, and even less about how they might develop, or how they interact in a developing mechanism. We have no substantial data on what level of development of specific aspects of processing might be achieved at a developmental stage (although we have general supportive information about memory and vocabulary development, for instance) and this seriously compromises our ability to construct appropriate intervention programmes.

Since the application of developmental cognitive neuropsychology is in its infancy, it is not surprising to see terms borrowed from the adult-acquired field. Bryan (1995) asks, with respect to developmental language and speech disorders, 'not just what are the errors but why did they occur and 'where' might the difficulties in processing be'. But to conceptualise developmental disorders as a series of errors is surely in itself incompatible with a notion of a developing organism. One cannot say that a child has made a semantic substitution error if they have never had the knowledge of that vocabulary. One might be able to say that the child has made an error of lexical retrieval, if they know the word (i.e. can comprehend it and produce it on other occasions) but substitute it with a related word on a word-naming task. So certain types of developmental language deficit seem to lend themselves more readily to analysis in a language processing model than others. This may appear a major obstacle for cognitive neuropsychology, but this is not necessarily the case. Developmental cognitive neuropsychology as a framework for intervention with circumscribed language deficits may have a substantial contribution to make. It is less likely to be of benefit where the deficits are widespread or where there are additional social and cognitive factors. A further limitation is that the nature of some assessments used also require a level of metalinguistic awareness which will not be present in the preschool child.

A further disadvantage underlines the bottom-up nature of the developmental cognitive neuropsychological approach. Most tasks within the model that are designed to 'tap' processes (the 'tapping' tasks) are based on single word activities. Doubtless there will be efforts made to extend the model to larger units of processing, but this does not satisfy the criticisms coming from the top-down approach. A child develops and uses language not in a single-word or single-sentence vacuum, but in an environment rich with linguistic and physical context, which provides support for communication and for learning about communication. Sarno, writing about acquired aphasia states '...scores on linguistic and neuropsychological measures may identify specific deficits which may or may not correlate with use of language for communication in everyday life' (Sarno, 1993). Context is a difficult concept to marry with cognitive neuropsychological models of language processing. Context also provides an invaluable variable in the therapeutic process, which is often under-used. Moreover, there is substantial evidence regarding the interaction between linguistic levels: where can this be accounted for in the model? Bryan cautions that 'it may not be possible to use this approach with every child'. We would argue, in the present state of knowledge, that the proportion of children with developmental language disorders for whom this approach could be used is limited, but that for the few who will benefit, the model may provide a clear rationale for therapy, from which not only the child, but also the clinician will gain.

Integration and eclecticism

It is conceivable that in the future, methods of intervention that combine the top-down and bottom-up approaches will begin to emerge. Gillam, McFadden and Van Kleeck (1995) describe an early example of such an integrated approach, when they outline the combination of 'Whole Language' and 'Language Skills' approaches in intervention for narrative skills in language-impaired children.

Both of the major approaches that we have outlined here are under-evaluated. By inference it would appear that top-down approaches lend themselves well to working with pragmatics and narrative abilities, but might be of less serviceability with, say, phonological impairments (Alcorn et al., 1995). Bottom-up approaches lend themselves especially well to intervention where the unit of language of interest (generally a phonological string) is more easily identifiable. As Ellis Weismer affirms, 'What seems most important is not which theoretical model is adopted but that a coherent conceptual framework is consistently employed to guide intervention efforts and related research questions' (Ellis Weismer, 1991).

We have laboured in the description of these two types of approaches

for two reasons. Firstly they demonstrate that progress is being made in
the discipline of intervention strategies and models. From disparate
routes, maybe, but they are nevertheless, emerging. The challenge for
the coming years is not to fall into the trap of blanket uninformed acceptance of new therapies but to adopt a critical approach to evaluation of
intervention. We should, as clinicians in the next millennium, be making
more informed choices because there will be a greater variety of therapies available that have been extensively investigated. To embrace fash-
ionable therapies without scepticism is a retrograde step. It remains
indisputably the case that the successful and satisfied clinician is usually
one who recognises that eclecticism is imperative when dealing with the
complex interaction of factors and individual variations in developmental language disorders.

What happens to these children?

In an attempt to redress the neglect of former years, attention is now
increasingly being directed to the long-term outcome for children with
developmental language impairments. The association between early
language delay and disorder and subsequent learning disability is very
strong (Strominger and Bashir, 1977; Aram and Nation, 1980; Silva,
McGee and Williams, 1983; Snowling, 1987; Tallal, 1987). Longitudinal
studies (e.g. Bishop and Adams, 1990) have shown convincing evidence
for the consequences of early language impairment on reading comprehension skills and other studies. (Paul and Cohen, 1984; Stone, 1992)
have demonstrated that the consequences of early deficits reach far into
the social and emotional domains, which in turn have a negative impact
on educational progress.

There are very good reasons to continue investigating language
disorders on the lines indicated above. Among the most cogent is the
hope that such investigations will result in better understanding and
more effective management. If children's difficulties can be identified
early and the course of the condition predicted, remedy can be chan-
nelled in the most efficient way. Studies to date have shown that there
is a core of language-disordered children who go on to become
learning disabled. Whether specialist intervention at one level can
result in reduction of impairment at another remains speculative. The
effects of therapy in altering the course of a language disorder have not
been measured in large numbers because the course of language disorders is only now starting to be clarified. Investigators to date have been
unable to affirm the positive effects of therapy in predicting outcome.
Bishop and Edmundson (1987a, b) are among those authors wishing
to make it clear that strong conclusions about therapy effectiveness
should not be drawn from their findings on this point. Their emphasis
is proper and thoughtful because speech and language therapy in the

UK has suffered from well-intentioned but premature attempts to evaluate its effectiveness. There is the need to be accountable and to be seen to be accountable, which is recognised by the whole profession. The public must be assured that the help given to the handicapped, help that costs the public money, is the most effective that can be devised. Speech and language therapists are under the obligation to reduce the effects of any potentially handicapping condition to the greatest extent possible. They are not, however, under the obligation to cure conditions which arise from some essential flaw in the mechanism. Society does not require this of those who practise medicine nor should it require it of those who work in the remedial and caring professions. What society does require is skilled and expert treatment from professionals that will help individual sufferers to realise their potential, compensate for their handicaps and live happily with themselves. The community must play a full part then in the social adjustment of the handicapped population. It will be easier for society to do this when professionals are more fully committed to a proselytising role on behalf of their clientele. Because this must stem from knowledge and commitment rather than emotional appeal, we are brought back to the need for clear thinking, comprehensive description and accurate prediction.

Individual speech and language therapists who have practised for many years have tried to find out what has happened to the young language-disordered children with whom they worked. In the case of one of the authors of this text (BBB), the search has been conducted on both sides of the Atlantic. There is, of course, a great variation in the success and happiness the children have experienced. Among the observations reported by parents and friends, the following tend to reoccur. 'He doesn't have many friends, I would describe him as a loner'. 'He doesn't have a girl friend yet; I think girls find him rather immature.' Sometimes therapists are able to observe for themselves behaviour that brings home to them the full extent of 'residual disabilities' they may have been inclined to dismiss. A spouse may report that someone has telephoned but the message was difficult to understand. The caller turns out to be one of the best graduates from the language unit. Or, watching an adolescent girl dancing at a party may suddenly reveal the full extent of her motor coordination difficulties. Signs of fatigue remind one of how tiring it must be to spend the whole day concentrating hard to pick up information that most of us gather in passing. A mother speaks of the tantrums her 20-year-old son will still display if interrupted whilst watching television because he will not then be able to understand what is happening. These are the kinds of deficits shown by the language-disordered population that distinguishes it far more effectively from the low-verbal section of the normal population than do broad measures of verbal ability (Snyder, 1982).

As our knowledge of language disorder increases, it is to be hoped that it will have a more pronounced and positive impact upon the flexible and continuous nature of service provision. In the meantime, it is important to prevent administrators from pinning provision to specific diagnoses or test results because these may be no better guides than the thoughtful results of experienced personnel. A final responsibility of professionals towards their clients is to make as sure as they can that professional services are employed to maximum advantage.

Conclusions

The views we have expressed regarding the nature of language disorders coupled with the likelihood that resources will show little appreciable growth in the immediate future give cause for a consideration, albeit speculative, about the direction speech and language therapy may follow within the next decade. We have seen a move away form the well worn pattern of once weekly, one to one therapy sessions to different models of delivery of service. Further changes await the investigation of the benefits of alternative regimes. Studies such as that of Kot and Law (1995), for instance, who compared the effects of two different types of treatment (group treatment with or without parental support), are of particular value. At the heart of such change we see a need for a radical reappraisal of selection criteria. Allied to this is the need for speech and language therapists to identify the nature of their specific knowledge and skills; i.e. those that are unique to them and not shared with parallel professional workers. Van der Gaag and Davies (1994) have provided valuable information on the special skills of speech and language therapists working with one client group.

There still, however, remains a core of children with intractable impairment who require concentrated specialised help, which will involve the therapist in detailed planning, and which will call upon a unique combination of knowledge derived from developmental psychology, neurobiological development and from applied linguistic science. For such children, rigid adherence to a pre-packaged language programme is unlikely to be helpful, for the intervention must be individually planned. The main advantage of such programmes is that, provided they are not over-prescriptive, they offer a common meeting ground and a guideline for cooperative effort between therapists and others. Over the last decade or so there has been a shift of focus on to those aspects of language that are more particularly concerned with communication and this is welcome. But our enthusiasm for pragmatic proficiency should not make us overlook the fact that those children with severe language disorder have no tools with which to demonstrate their ability to use language. For these, work must begin at the 'coal face' of structure and meaning. It is in this sphere that we consider speech and language therapists to possess special expertise.

In relation to developmental language disorders there seem to be three main areas in which speech and language therapists' work is still developing.

- In the first instance there needs to be a concentration and application of therapeutic skills for the benefit of severely language-impaired children.
- Cooperative work with parents both in devising and monitoring their work must be encouraged to a much greater extent. The advent of the Hanen programme has accelerated the process of parent education and work on managing parent–child interactions is increasingly reported in the literature (Kelman and Schneider, 1994).
- We need to be aware of the special contribution that teachers are able to make, especially in those cases where learning difficulties and language problems coexist. To this end teachers must have the opportunity to learn about the nature of disordered language whilst therapists in turn also need to become more familiar with the ways in which teachers seek to help those with learning difficulties. Work is now being done to bring the two professions closer together through training and collaboration in schools (Newman, 1996; Wright, 1996).

But precisely because there is much current uncertainty and ever greater discovery still to be made in the future about the nature of language disorders, we strongly advocate a flexible approach. Knowledge accrues as more research is carried out; the thoughts and views in this updated text have been influenced by the research of the last ten years, and doubtless a book written ten years hence would differ from this text substantially, as insight and discernment grow.

References

Abudarham S (1987) Fact and fiction. In S Abudarham (Ed.) Bilingualism and the Bilingual. Windsor: NFER-Nelson.

Adams C (1990) Syntactic comprehension in children with expressive language impairment. British Journal of Disorders of Communication 25: 149–72.

Adams C, Bishop DVM (1989) Conversational characteristics of children with semantic–pragmatic language disorder. I: Exchange structure, turntaking, repairs and cohesion. British Journal of Disorders of Communication 24: 211–39

Adams C, Conti-Ramsden G (1995) Developmental language disorders. In Grundy K (Ed.) Linguistics in Clinical Practice (Second Edn). London: Whurr.

AFASIC (1988) Language Unit Guidelines. 347 Central Markets, London EC1A 9NH.

AFASIC (1991) The AFASIC Checklists. Wishbech: LDA.

Alcorn M, Jarratt T, Martin W, Dodd B (1995) Intensive group therapy: Efficacy of a whole-language approach. In Dodd B (Ed.) The Differential Diagnosis and Treatment of Children with Speech Disorder. London: Whurr.

Aldred C (1983) Language in use. Bulletin of College of Speech Therapists, London; October.

Allen GD, Hawkins S (1978) The development of phonological rhythm. In Bell A, Hooper D (Eds) Syllables and Segments. Amsterdam: North Holland.

Aram D, Nation J (1975) Patterns of language behavior in children with developmental language disorders. Journal of Speech and Hearing Research 18: 229–41.

Aram D, Nation J (1980) Preschool language disorders and subsequent language and academic difficulties. Journal of Communicative Disorders 13: 159–70.

Aram D, Nation J (1982) Child Language Disorders, St Louis, MO: CV Mosby.

Aram DM, Hack M, Hawkins S, Weissman BM, Borawaski-Clark E (1991) Very-low-birthweight children and speech and language development. Journal of Speech and Hearing Research 34: 1169–79.

Baker L (1988) The use of language sample analysis. Bulletin of College of Speech Therapists, May.

Barrows HS, Pickell GC (1991) Developing Clinical Problem Solving Skills. New York/London: Norton and Co.

Bartak L, Rutter M, Cox A (1975) A comparative study of infantile autism and specific developmental language disorders. British Journal of Psychiatry 126: 127–45.

Bath D (1981) Developing the speech therapy service in day nurseries: A progress report. British Journal of Disorders of Communication 16: 159–74.

Bax M (1987) Paediatric assessment of the child with a speech and language disorder. In Yule W, Rutter M (Eds) Language Development and Disorders. Oxford: SIMP, Blackwell Scientific and Lippincott.

Bax M, Hart H, Jenkins S (1980) Assessment of speech and language development in the young child. Pediatrics 66: 350–4.

Beech J, Harding L, Hilton-Jones D (1993) Assessment in speech and language therapy. London: Routledge.

Beitcham JH, Nair R, Clegg M, Patel PG (1986) Prevalence of speech and language disorders in five-year-old kindergarten children in the Ottowa–Carleton region. Journal of Speech and Hearing Disorders 51: 98–119.

Bellugi U, Marks S, Bihrle A, Sabo H (1993) Dissociation between language and cognitive functions in Williams Syndrome. In Bishop D, Mogford K (Eds) Language Development in Exceptional Circumstances. Hove: Lawrence Erlbaum Associates.

Benton AL (1964) Developmental aphasia and brain damage. Cortex 1: 40–52.

Benton A (1978) The cognitive functioning of children with developmental dysphasia. In Wyke M (Ed.) Developmental Dysphasia. London: Academic Press.

Berndt R S, Mitchum CC (1995) Cognitive neuropsychological approaches to the treatment of language disorders. Hove: Lawrence Erlbaum Associates.

Bernhardt B, Gilbert J (1992) Applying linguistic theory to speech–language pathology: the case for nonlinear phonology. Clinical Linguistics and Phonetics 6: 123–45.

Berger M (1987) What is a language disorder? Proceedings of First International Symposium Specific Speech and Language Disorders in Children, University of Reading. London: AFASIC.

Berry MF (1969) Language Disorders of Children. New York: Appleton-Century-Crofts.

Berry MF (1980) Teaching Linguistically Handicapped Children. Englewood Cliffs, NJ: Prentice-Hall.

Beveridge M, Conti-Ramsden G (1987) Children with Language Disabilities. Milton Keynes: Open University Press.

Bishop DVM (1979) Comprehension in developmental language disorders. Developmental Medicine and Child Neurology 21: 225–38.

Bishop DVM (1983) Comprehension of English syntax by profoundly deaf children. Journal of Child Psychology and Psychiatry 24: 415–34.

Bishop DVM (1985) Age at onset and outcome in 'Acquired Aphasia and Convulsive Disorder' (Landau–Kleffner syndrome). Developmental Medicine and Child Neurology 27: 705–12.

Bishop DVM (1986) Some new data using the EPVT (full range version with a British sample) British Journal of Disorders of Communication 21: 209–21.

Bishop DVM (1987a) The causes of specific developmental language disorder (developmental dysphasia). Journal of Child Psychology and Psychiatry 28: 1–8.

Bishop DVM (1987b) The concept of comprehension in language disorders. Proceedings of First International Symposium Specific Speech and Language Disorders in Children, University of Reading. London: AFASIC.

Bishop DVM (1989) Autism, Asperger's syndrome and semantic-pragmatic disorder: where are the boundaries? British Journal of Disorders of Communication 24: 107–21.

Bishop DVM (1990) Handedness, clumsiness and developmental language disorders. Neuropsychologia 28: 681–90.

Bishop DVM (1992a) The biological basis of specific language impairment. In Fletcher P, Hall D (Eds) Specific Speech and Language Disorders in Children. London: Whurr.

Bishop DVM (1992b) The underlying nature of specific language impairment. Journal of Child Psychology and Psychiatry 33: 3–66.

Bishop DVM (1994) Grammatical errors in specific language impairment: competence or performance limitations? Applied Psycholinguistics 15: 507–50.

Bishop DVM, Adams C (1989) Conversational characteristics of children with semantic–pragmatic language disorder. II: What features lead to a judgement of inappropriacy? British Journal of Disorders of Communication 24: 241–63.

Bishop DVM, Adams C (1990) A prospective study of the relationship between specific language impairment, phonological disorder and reading retardation. Journal of Child Psychology and Psychiatry 31: 1027–50.

Bishop DVM, Adams C (1991) What do referential communication tasks measure? A study of children with specific language impairment. Applied Psycholinguistics 1: 225–78.

Bishop DVM, Edmundson A (1986) Is otitis media a major cause of developmental language disorders? British Journal of Disorders of Communication 21: 321–38.

Bishop DVM, Edmundson A (1987a) Language-impaired 4-year-olds. Distinguishing transient from persistent impairment. Journal of Speech and Hearing Disorders 52: 156–73.

Bishop DVM, Edmundson A (1987b) Specific language impairment as a maturational lag: evidence from longitudinal data on language and motor development. Developmental Medicine and Child Neurology 29: 442–49.

Bishop DVM, Rosenbloom L (1987) Childhood language disorders. Classification and overview. In Yule W, Rutter M (Eds) Language Development and Disorders. Oxford: SIMP, Blackwell Scientific and Lippincott.

Bishop DVM, Byers Brown B, Robson J (1990) The relationship between phoneme discrimination, speech production and language comprehension in cerebral-palsied individuals. Journal of Speech and Hearing Research 33: 210–19.

Blank M, Marquis MA (1987) Directing Discourse. Tucson, AZ: Communication Skill Builders.

Bloom L (1973) One Word at a Time. The Use of Single-word Utterances Before Syntax. The Hague: Mouton.

Bloom L, Lahey M (1978) Language Development and Language Disorders. New York: John Wiley.

Boomer DS, Laver J (1968). Slips of the tongue. British Journal of Disorders of Communication 3: 2–12.

Bortolini U, Leonard LB (1991) The speech of phonologically disordered children acquiring Italian. Clinical Linguistics and Phonetics 5: 1–12.

Bridgeman E, Snowling M (1988) The perception of phoneme sequence: a comparison of dyspraxic and normal children. British Journal of Disorders of Communication 23: 245–52.

Broadbent D (1958) Perception and Communication. Oxford: Pergamon.

Brown A (1975) The development of memory. In Reese H (Ed.) Advances in Child Development and Behaviour. New York: Academic Press.

Brown R (1973) A First Language. The Early Stages. Cambridge, MA: Harvard University Press.

Brown R, Berko J (1960) Word association and the acquisition of grammar. Child Development 31: 1–14.

Browning EF (1987) I Can't See What You Are Saying. London: Angel Press.

Bruner J (1975) The ontogenesis of speech acts. Journal of Child Language 2: 1–15.

Bruner J (1983a) Child's Talk. New York: W.W. Norton.

Bruner J (1983b) In Search of Mind. New York: Harper and Row.

Bryan A (1995) Boxes and arrows for children. Bulletin of the Royal College of Speech and Language Therapists, November, 14–16.

Bryan A, Howard D (1992) Frozen phonology thawed: the analysis and remediation of a developmental disorder of real word phonology. European Journal of Disorders of Communication 27: 343–65.

Bryan A, North C (1994) Developmental cognitive neuropsychology: a comparison of two case studies. Child Language Teaching and Therapy 10: 313–27.

Bryant P (1985) The question of prevention. In Snowling M (Ed.) Children's Written Language Difficulties. Windsor: NFER-Nelson.

Butler D (1987) Cushla and Her Books. Harmondsworth: Penguin.

Butler D (1988) Babies Need Books. Harmondsworth: Penguin.

Butler KRG (1984). Language processing. Half way up the down staircase. In Wallach GP, Butler KG (Eds) Language Learning Disabilities in School Age Children. Baltimore, MD: Williams and Wilkins.

Byers Brown B (1971) A suggested rationale for the treatment of developmental disorders of language. In Perrin GE, Trim JL (Eds) Applications of Linguistics, Selected papers of the Second International Conference of Applied Linguistics, Cambridge.

Byers Brown B (1976) Language vulnerability, speech delay and therapeutic intervention. British Journal of Diseases of Communication 11: 43–56.

Byers Brown B (1981) Speech Therapy. Principles and Practice. Edinburgh: Churchill Livingstone.

Byers Brown B (1982) Clinical factors in language disorder: Core implicit and crisis induced. Paper presented at Annual Convention of American Speech, Language and Hearing Association, Toronto, Canada.

Byers Brown B (1985) Evidence upon which to act: The identification of communication disorders. Jansson Memorial Lecture London. British Journal of Disorders of Communication 20: 3–18.

Byers Brown B (1987) Early identification of language disorders. Proceedings of First International Symposium Specific Speech and Language Disorders in Children, University of Reading. London: AFASIC.

Byers Brown B (1988) The utterances of one-year-old infants. Proceedings of Child Language Conference, University of Warwick.

Byers Brown B, Beveridge M (1979) Language Disorders in Children, Monograph, No. 1. London: College of Speech Therapists.

Byers Brown B, Lewis M (1984) Speech–sound behaviour at one year of age. Proceedings of Symposium on Research in Child Language Disorders, University of Wisconsin, Madison, WI.

Byers Brown B, Bendersky M, Chapman T (1986) The early utterances of preterm infants. British Journal of Disorders of Communication 21: 307–20.

Campbell RN (1979) Cognitive development and child language. In Fletcher P, Garman M (Eds) Language Acquisition. Cambridge: Cambridge University Press.

Cantwell D, Baker L (1987) Developmental Speech and Language Disorders. New York: Guilford Press.

Cantwell D, Baker L, Rutter M (1978) A comparative study of infantile autism and specific developmental receptive language disorder–IV. Analysis of syntax and language function. Journal of Child Psychology and Psychiatry 19: 351–62

Capute AJ, Palmer FB, Shapiro BK, Wachtel RG, Schmidt S, Ross A (1986) Clinical and auditory milestone scale: Prediction of cognition in infancy. Developmental Medicine and Child Neurology 28: 762–71.

Caramazza A, Zurif EB (1978) Comprehension of center embedded sentences in aphasia and in development. In: The Development and Breakdown of Language Functions. Parallels and Divergencies. Baltimore, MD: The Johns Hopkins Press.

Chiat S, Hirson A (1987) From conceptual intention to utterance: a study of impaired language output in a child with developmental dysphasia. British Journal of Disorders of Communication 22: 37–64.

Chiat S, Hunt J (1993) Connections between phonology and semantics: an exploration of lexical processing in a language-impaired child. Child Language Teaching and Therapy 9: 200–13.

Chomsky N (1986) Knowledge of Language: Its Nature, Origin and Use. New York: Praeger.

Clahsen H (1989) The grammatical characterisation of developmental dysphasia. Linguistics 27: 897–920.

Cole KN, Dale PS, Mills PE. (1990) Defining language delay in young children by cognitive referencing: Are we saying more than we know? Applied Psycholinguistics 11: 291–302.

Cole KN, Schwartz IS, Notari AR, Dale PS, Mills PE (1995) Examination of the stability of two methods of defining specific language impairment. Applied Psycholinguistics 16: 103–23.

College of Speech and Language Therapists (1990) Communicating Quality. London: College of Speech and Language Therapists.

College of Speech Therapists (1988a) Position paper: The role of speech therapists in child language disability. London: College of Speech Therapists.

College of Speech Therapists (1988b) Position paper 2/88: Education Act 1981, Guidelines for Speech Therapists. London: College of Speech Therapists.

Coltheart M (1987) Producing language. In Harris M, Coltheart M (Eds) Language Processing in Children and Adults. London: Routledge, Keegan and Paul.

Coltheart M, Job, Sartori G (1988) The cognitive neuropsychology of language. Hove: Lawrence Erlbaum Associates.

Conti-Ramsden G (1987) Mother–child talk with language-impaired children Proceedings of First International Symposium Specific Speech and Language Disorders in Children, University of Reading. London: AFASIC.

Conti-Ramsden G (1990) Maternal recasts and other contingent replies to language-impaired children. Journal of Speech and Hearing Disorders 55: 262–74.

Conti-Ramsden G (1993) Using parents to foster communicatively-impaired children's language development. Seminars in Speech and Language 14: 289–95

Conti-Ramsden G, Gunn C (1986) The development of conversational disability: a case study. British Journal of Disorders of Communication 21: 339–51.

Conti-Ramsden G, Dykins J (1991) Mother–child interactions with language impaired children and their siblings. British Journal of Disorders of Communication 17: 3–19.

Cooper JM (1985) Children with specific learning difficulties: the role of the speech therapist. In Snowling M (Ed.)Children's Written Language Difficulties. Windsor: NFER-Nelson.

Cooper JM, Griffiths CPS (1978) Treatment and prognosis in developmental dysphasia. In Wyke M (Ed.) Developmental Dysphasia. London: Academic Press.

Cooper JM, Moodley M, Reynell J (1978) Helping Language Development. London: Edward Arnold.

Coupe J, Goldbart J (1987) Communication Before Speech. Normal Development and Impaired Communication. London: Croom Helm.

Crago M, Gopnik M (1994) From families to phenotypes: theoretical and clinical implications of research into the genetic basis of specific language impairment. In

Watkins RV, Rice ML (Eds) Specific Language Impairments in Children. Baltimore, MD: Paul Brookes.

Craig F, Tulving E (1975) Depth of processing and retention of words in episodic memory. Journal of Experimental Psychology: General 104: 268–94.

Crary MA (1984) A neurolinguistic perspective of developmental dyspraxia. Communication Disorders 9: 3.

Crary MA (1993) Developmental Motor Speech Disorders. London: Whurr.

Creaghead NA, Newman PW, Secord WA (1989) Assessment and remediation of articulatory and phonological disorders (Second Edn) Columbus, OH: Merrill Publishing Company.

Crystal D (1981) Clinical Linguistics. Disorders of Communication. Vienna: Springer–Verlag.

Crystal D (1982a) Terms, time and teeth. British Journal of Disorders of Communication 17: 3–19.

Crystal D (1982b) Profiling Linguistic Disability. London: Edward Arnold.

Crystal D (1986) Listen to Your Child. Harmondsworth: Penguin.

Crystal D (1987) Towards a 'bucket' theory of language disability: taking account of interaction between linguistic levels. Clinical Linguistica and Phonetics 1: 2–7.

Crystal D, Fletcher P, Garman M (1976 and 1989) The Grammatical Analysis of Language Disability. (First and Second Edn). London: Edward Arnold.

Curtiss S (1977) Genie. A psycholinguistic study of a modern day wild child. London: Academic Press.

Curtiss S, Katz W, Tallal P (1992) Delay versus deviance in the language acquisition of language-impaired children. Journal of Speech and Hearing Research 35: 373–83.

Damico JS (1988) The lack of efficacy in language therapy. A case study. Language and Speech and Hearing Services in Schools 19: 41–50.

Dean E, Howell J, Hill A, Waters D (1990) Metaphon resource pack manual. Windsor: NFER- Nelson.

Dean E, Howell J, Waters D, Reid J (1995) Metaphon: a metalinguistic approach to the treatment of phonological disorders in children. Clinical Linguistics and Phonetics 9: 1–58.

Del Priore C, Valance S, Day R (1987) Understanding the communication disordered child: a developmental and observational perspective. Proceedings of First International Symposium: Specific Speech and Language Disorders in Children, University of Reading. London: AFASIC.

Dixon J, Kot A, Law J (1988) Early language screening in City and Hackney: work in progress. Child Care, Health and Development 14: 213–29.

Dobbing J (1972) Growth of the brain. In: Science Journal. The Human Brain. London: Paladin

Dodd B (1995) Differential diagnosis and treatment of children with speech disorder. London: Whurr.

Dollaghan CA Campbell TF (1992) A procedure for classifying disruptions in spontaneous language samples. Topics in Language Disorders 12: 56–68.

Donahue M (1987) Interaction between linguistic and pragmatic development in learning disabled children: three views of the state of the union. In Rosenberg S (Ed.) Advances in Applied Psycholinguistics, Vol. 1. Cambridge: Cambridge University Press.

Doswell G, Lewis V, Sylva K, Boucher J (1994) Validation data on the Warwick Symbolic Play Test. European Journal of Disorders of Communication 29: 289–98.

Douglass RL (1983) Defining and describing clinical accountability. Seminars in Speech and Language 4: 107–18.

Duggirala V, Dodd B (1991) A psycholinguistic assessment model for disordered phonology. In: Congress of Phonetic Sciences, Aix-en-Provence, Université de Provence, pp. 342–45.

Edwards JR (1979) Language and Disadvantage. London: Edward Arnold.

Edwards M (1982) Verbal dyspraxia: a disorder of rhythm and seriation. Unpublished pilot study.

Edwards M (1984) Disorders of Articulation: Aspects of Dysarthria and Dyspraxia Disorders of Communication. Vienna: Springer–Verlag.

Edwards M, Brown N, Cape J, Foreman D (1984) Criteria for selection of children for speech therapy. Unpublished report. Funded by Department of Health and Social Services.

Eisenson J (1972) Aphasia in Children. New York: Harper and Row.

Eisenson J (1985) Central auditory disorders and developmental aphasia. Is there a difference? Human Communication (Canada) 9: 13–16.

Eisenson J (1986) Developmental (congenital) aphasia and acquired aphasia and dysphasia. Human Communication (Canada) 10: 5–9.

Ellis AW, Young AW (1988) Human cognitive neuropsychology. Hove: Lawrence Erlbaum Associates.

Ellis Robinson MR (1987) Provision and management for primary speech and language disorders in Australia. Proceedings of First International Symposium. Specific Speech and Language Disorders in Children. University of Reading. London: AFASIC.

Ellis Weismer S (1991) Child language intervention: research issues on the horizon. In Miller J (Ed.) Research on Child Language Disorders. Texas: Pro-ed.

Ellis Weismer S, Murray-Branch J, Miller JF (1994) A prospective longitudinal study of language development in late talkers. Journal of Speech and Hearing Research 37: 852–67.

Enderby P, Davies P (1989) Communication disorders: Planning a service to meet the needs. British Journal of Disorders of Communication 24: 301–331.

Enderby P, Emerson J (1995) Does Speech and Language Therapy Work? A Review of the Literature. London: Whurr.

Faucett GF, Clibbons JS (1983) The acquisition of signs by the mentally handicapped. British Journal of Disorders of Communication 18: 13–21.

Fey ME (1986) Language Intervention with Young Children. San Diego,CA: College Hill Press.

Fey ME, Catts HW, Larrivee LS (1995) Preparing preschoolers for the academic and social challenges of school. In Fey ME, Windsor J, Warren SF (Eds) Language Intervention: Preschool Through the Elementary Years. Baltimore, MD: Paul Brookes.

Flavell JH, Miller PH, Miller S (1993) Cognitive Development, (Third Edn). Englewood Cliffs, NJ: Prentice Hall .

Fletcher P (1987) The basis of language impairment in children: a comment on Chiat and Hirson. British Journal of Disorders of Communication 22: 65–72.

Fletcher P (1991) Subgroups in school-age language impaired children. In Fletcher P, Hall D (Eds) Specific Speech and Language Disorders in Children. London: Whurr.

Fletcher P (1992) Lexical verbs and language impairment: a case study. Clinical Linguistics and Phonetics 6: 147–54.

Frankenburg WK, Fandal AW, Sciarelto W, Burgess D (1981) The newly abbreviated and revised Denver Developmental Screening Test. Journal of Pediatrics 33: 335–99.

Fundudis T, Kolvin I, Garside R (1979) Speech Retarded and Deaf Children. London: Academic Press.

Furrow D, Nelson K (1986) Another look at the motherese hypothesis: a reply to Gleitman. Journal of Child Language 13: 153–67.

Gallagher TM (1983) Pre-assessment. A procedure for accommodating language use variability. In Gallagher TM, Prutting CA (Eds) Pragmatic Assessment and Intervention. San Diego, CA: College Hill Press.

Gardner H (1994) Doing talk about speech: a study of phonologically disordered children and speech therapists working together. Unpublished doctoral thesis; University of York.

Gardner H (1995) Are your minimal pairs too neat? Paper given at the Golden Jubilee Conference of the Royal College of Speech Therapists, York.

Garrett MF (1980) Levels of processing in sentence production. In Butterworth B (Ed.) Language Production, Vol. 1. London: Academic Press.

Garvey M, Mutton DE (1973) Sex chromosome aberrations and speech development. Archives of the Disturbed Child 48: 937–41.

Garvey C, Kramer TL (1988) The language of social pretend play. Unpublished paper.

Gathercole S (1994) Word learning in language-impaired children. Child Language Teaching and Therapy 9: 187–99.

Gathercole SE, Baddeley AD (1989) Development of vocabulary in children depends upon short term phonological memory. Journal of Memory and Language 28: 200–213.

Gathercole SE, Baddeley AD (1990) Phonological memory deficits in language disordered children. Is there a causal connection? Journal of Memory and Language 29: 336–360.

Gathercole SE, Baddeley AD (1993) Working Memory and Language. Hove: Lawrence Erlbaum Associates.

Gerard K (1986) The checklist of communicative competence. Available from the author at 3 Perry Mansions, 113 Catford Hill, London SE 6.

German DJ (1985) The use of specific semantic word categories in the diagnosis of dysnomic learning-disabled children. British Journal of Disorders of Communication 20: 143–54.

German DJ (1987) Spontaneous language profiles of children with word finding problems. Language Speech and Hearing Services in Schools 18: 206–16.

German D J (1992) Word finding intervention for children and adolescents. Topics in Language Disorders 13: 33–50.

German D, Simon E (1991) Analysis of children's word-finding skills in discourse. Journal of Speech and Hearing Research 34: 309–16

Geschwind N, Levitsky W (1968) Human brain: left–right asymmetries in the temporal speech region. Science 161: 186–87.

Gibbon F, Grunwell P (1992) Specific developmental language learning disabilities. In Grunwell P (Ed.) Developmental Speech Disorders. London: Whurr.

Gibson D, Ingram D (1983) The onset of comprehension in a language delayed child. Applied Psycholinguistics 4: 359–70.

Gillam R, McFadden TU, Van Kleeck A (1995) Improving narrative abilities: Whole language and language skills approaches. In Fey ME, Windsor J, Warren SF (Eds) Language Intervention: Preschool Through the Elementary Years. Baltimore, MD: Paul Brookes.

Gleitman L, Newport C, Gleitman H (1984) The current state of the motherese hypothesis. Journal of Child Language 11: 43–79.

Glogowska M (1996) A step in the right direction. Bulletin of the Royal College of Speech and Language Therapists, April, 16–17.

Golinkoff RM (1983) The preverbal negotiation of failed messages: insights into the transition period. In Golinkoff RM (Ed.) The Transition from Prelinguistic to Linguistic Communication. Hillsdale, NJ: Lawrence Erlbaum.

Goodman R (1987) The developmental neurobiology of language. In Yule W, Rutter M (Eds) Language Development and Disorders. Oxford: SIMP, Blackwell Scientific and Lippincott.

Gopnik A (1988) Three types of early word: the emergence of social words, names and cognitive–relational words in the one word stage of development. First Language 8: 49–70.

Gopnik M (1990) Feature blindness: a case study. Language Acquisition 1: 139–64.

Gopnik M, Crago MB (1991) Familial aggregation of a developmental language disorder. Cognition 39: 1–50.

Gordon N (1966) The child who does not talk. Problems of diagnosis with special reference to children with severe auditory agnosia. British Journal of Disorders of Communication 1: 78–84.

Gordon N (1987) Developmental disorders of language. In Yule W, Rutter M (Eds) Language Development and Disorders. Oxford: SIMP, Blackwell Scientific and Lippincott.

Gordon N, McKinlay I (1980) Helping Clumsy Children. Edinburgh: Churchill Livingstone.

Gravel JS, Wallace IF (1992) Listening and language at 4 years of age: effects of early otitis media. Journal of Speech and Hearing Research 35: 588–95.

Greene MCL (1963) A comparison of children with delayed speech due to coordination disorder or language learning difficulty. Speech Pathology and Therapy 6: 69–77.

Greene MCL (1964) Differential diagnosis of developmental aphasia. Speech Pathology and Therapy 7: 84–93.

Griffiths CPS (1964) Treatment of developmental aphasia. Speech Pathology and Therapy 7: 95–99.

Griffiths CPS (1969) A follow-up study of children with disorders of speech. British Journal of Disorders of Communication 4: 46–56.

Griffiths CPS (1972) Developmental Aphasia: An Introduction. London: ICAA (now ICAN).

Grundy K (1995a) Developmental Speech Disorders. In Grundy K (Ed.) Linguistics in Clinical Practice (2nd Edn). London: Taylor and Francis.

Grundy K (1995b) Metaphon: unique and effective? Clinical Linguistics and Phonetics 9: 20 –24.

Grunwell P (1975) The phonological analysis of language disorders. British Journal of Disorders of Communication 10: 1–31.

Grunwell P (1980a) Developmental language disorders at the phonological level. In Jones M (Ed.) Language Disabilities in Children. Lancaster: MTP Press.

Grunwell P (1980b) Procedures for child assessment: a review. British Journal of Disorders of Communication 15: 189–203.

Grunwell P (1981) The Nature of Phonological Disability in Children. London: Academic Press.

Grunwell P (1982) Clinical Phonology. London: Croom Helm.

Grunwell P, Russell J (1987) Vocalisations before, and after cleft palate surgery: a pilot study. British Journal of Disorders of Communication 22: 1–18.

Gubbay SS (1975) The Clumsy Child. Philadelphia, PA: WB Saunders.

Guralnick MJ, Bennett PC (Eds) (1987) The framework for early intervention. In: The Effectiveness of Early Intervention for At-risk and Handicapped Children. New York: Academic Press.

Hall D (1991) Health for All Children. Oxford: Oxford University Press.

Hall D (1992) Early screening and intervention. In Fletcher P, Hall D (Eds) Specific Speech and Language Disorders in Children: Correlates, Characteristics and Outcomes. London: Whurr.

Halliday MAK (1963) The Tones of English. Archives of Linguistics 15: 1–28.

Halliday MAK (1975) Learning How to Mean. Explorations in the Development of Language. London: Edward Arnold.

Hamilton P, Owrid HL (1974) Comparison of hearing impairment and sociocultural disadvantage in relation to verbal retardation. British Journal of Audiology 8: 27–32.

Harris J (1984) Teaching children to develop language: the impossible dream. In Miller D (Ed.) Remediating Children's Language. Behavioural and Naturalistic Approaches. London: Croom Helm.

Harris M, Coltheart M (1986) Language Processing in Children and Adults: An Introduction. London: Routledge, Keegan and Paul.

Hasenstab SM (1987) Language Learning and Otitis Media. London: Taylor and Francis.

Haynes C (1986) Assessment for identification and for therapy. In Advances in Working with Language-disordered Children. ICAN Conference Proceedings, London.

Haynes C, Naidoo S (1991) Children with specific speech and language impairment. Oxford: MacKeith Press.

Health for All Children (1989) Report of Joint Working Party Preschool Child Surveillance. Oxford: Medical Publications.

Hebb DO (1972) Textbook of Psychology, (Third Edn). Philadelphia, PA: WB Saunders.

Hitch GJ, Halliday MS (1983) Working memory in children. Philosophical Transactions of the Royal Society 302: 325–40.

Howard L, Hesketh A (1993) Metaphon: from effectiveness to efficiency. Bulletin of the College of Speech and Language Therapists, December.

Howard S, Hartley J, Muller D (1995) The changing face of child language assessment 1985–1995. Child Language Teaching and Therapy 11: 6–22.

Howell J, Dean E (1987) I think that's a noisy sound: reflection and learning in the therapeutic situation. Child Language Teaching and Therapy 3: 259–66.

Howell J, Dean E (1994) Treating Phonological Disorders in Children: Metaphon-Theory into Practice. London: Whurr.

Howlin J, Kendall L (1991) Assessing children with language tests–which tests to use? British Journal of Disorders of Communication 26: 355–67.

Hubbell RD (1981) Children's Language Disorders. Englewood Cliffs, NJ: Prentice Hall.

Hutt E (1986) Teaching Language-disordered Children. A Structured Curriculum. London: Edward Arnold.

Hutt E, Donlan C (1987) Adequate provision? A survey of language units. London: ICAN.

Hyde Wright S (1993) Teaching word-finding strategies to severely language-impaired children. European Journal of Disorders of Communication 28: 165–75

Hyde Wright S, Cray B (1991) A teacher's and a speech therapist's approach to management. In Mogford-Bevan K, Sadler J (Eds) Child Language Disability II. Avon: Multilingual Matters.

ICAN (1988) Units for Primary School Children with Speech and Language Disorders. Suggested Guidelines. London: ICAN.

Ingram D (1974) Phonological rules in young children. Journal of Child Language 1: 49–64.

Ingram D (1976) Phonological Disability in Children. London: Edward Arnold.

Ingram D (1987) Categories of phonological disorder. Proceedings of First International Symposium Specific Speech and Language Disorders in Children, University of Reading. London: AFASIC.

Ingram TTS (1959) Specific developmental disorders of speech in childhood. Brain 82: 450–67.

Jerger S, Jerger J, Alford BR, Abrams S (1983) Development of speech intelligibility in children with recurrent otitis media. Ear and Hearing 4: 138–45.

Johnston J (1994) Cognitive abilities of children with language impairment. In Watkins RV, Rice ML (Eds) Specific Language Impairments in Children. Baltimore, MD: Paul Brookes.

Johnston J, Newport E (1989) Critical period effects in second language learning: The influence of maturational state on the acquisition of English as a second language. Cognitive Psychology 21: 60–9.

Johnston J, Smith LB (1989) Dimensional thinking in language-impaired children. Journal of Speech and Hearing Research 32: 33–8.

Kagan J (1971) Change and Continuity in Infancy. New York: John Wiley.

Kail R, Hale CA, Leonard LB, Nippold MA (1984) Lexical storage and retrieval in language-impaired children. Applied Psycholinguistics 9: 37–49.

Kamhi A (1985) Questioning the value of large numerical multivariate studies: a response to Schery. Journal of Speech and Hearing Disorders 50: 288–90.

Kamhi AG, Catts HW (1989) Reading disabilities: a developmental language perspective. Newton, MA: Allyn and Bacon.

Kamhi AG, Catts HW, Mauer D, Apel K, Gentry BF (1988) Phonological and spatial processing abilities in language and reading-impaired children. Journal of Speech and Hearing Disorders 53: 316–27.

Kellett B, Lee B, Mobley P (1984) The Kellett Colour Coding Scheme. Private publication, Central Manchester Health Authority.

Kelly J, Local J (1989) Doing Phonology. Manchester: Manchester University Press.

Kelman E, Schneider C (1994) Parent–child interaction: an alternative approach to the management of children's language difficulties. Child Language Teaching and Therapy 10: 81–95.

Kent RD (1984) Psychobiology of speech development: co-emergence of language and a movement system. American Journal of Physiology 246: 855–942.

King RR, Jones C, Lasky E (1982) In retrospect: a fifteen year follow-up report of speech and language-disordered children. Language, Speech and Hearing Services in Schools 13: 24–32.

Kirchner DM, Klatzky RL (1985) Verbal rehearsal and memory in language disordered children. Journal of Speech and Hearing Research 28: 556–65.

Kirk U (Ed.) (1983) Neuropsychology of Language, Reading and Spelling. London: Academic Press.

Kluppel D (1991) Needed: Intervention research. In Miller J (Ed.) Research on Child Language Disorders. Austin, TX: Pro-ed.

Kot A, Law J (1995) Intervention with preschool children with specific language impairments: a comparison of two different approaches to treatment. Child Language Teaching and Therapy 11: 144–62.

Lahey M (1990) Who shall be called language disordered? Some reflections and one perspective. Journal of Speech and Hearing Disorders 55: 612–20.

Lahey M, Edwards J (1995) Specific Language Impairment: Preliminary investigation of factors associated with family history and with patterns of language performance. Journal of Speech and Hearing Research 38: 643–57.

Largo RH, Howard JA (1979) Developmental progression in play behaviour of children between nine and thirty months: 2. Spontaneous play and language development. Developmental Medicine and Child Neurology 21: 492–503.

Lashley KS (1951) The problem of serial order in behaviour. In Jeffress LA (Ed.) Cerebral Mechanisms and Behavior. New York: John Wiley.

Law J (1992) The early identification of language impairment in children. London: Chapman and Hall.

Law J, Pollard C (1994) Identifying speech and language delay. Health Visitor 67: 59–60.

Lea J (1965) A language scheme for children suffering from receptive aphasia. Speech Pathology and Therapy 8: 58–68.

Lea J (1986) A follow-up study of severely speech and language handicapped school leavers. Paper presented at ICAN Conference Advances in Working with Language Disordered Children, London.

Lees J (1993) Children with Acquired Aphasias. London: Whurr.

Lees J, Urwin S (1991) Children with Language Disorders. London: Whurr.

Lenneberg E (1967) The Biological Foundation of Language. New York: John Wiley.

Leonard LB (1972) What is deviant language? Journal of Speech and Hearing Disorders 37: 427–46.

Leonard LB (1981) Facilitating language skills in children with specific language impairment. Applied Psycholinguistics 2: 89–118.

Leonard LB (1987) Is specific language disorder a useful construct? In Rosenberg S (Ed.) Advances in Applied Psycholinguistics, Vol. 1. Disorders of First Language Development. Cambridge: Cambridge University Press.

Leonard LB, Dromi E (1994) The use of Hebrew verb morphology by children with specific language impairment and children developing language normally. First Language 14: 283–304.

Leonard LB, Prutting C, Perozi J, Berkey RK (1978) Non standardised approaches to the assessment of language behavior. ASHA 209: 371–79.

Leonard LB, McGregor KK, Allen GG (1992) Grammatical morphology and speech perception in children with specific language impairment. Journal of Speech and Hearing Research 35: 1076–85.

Leonard LB, Sabbadini L, Leonard J, Volterra V (1987) Specific language impairment in children: a crosslinguistic study. Brain and Language 32: 233–52.

Letts C (1985) Linguistic interaction in the clinic: How do therapists do therapy? Child Language Teaching and Therapy 1: 321–31.

Letts C, Reid J (1994) Using conversational data in the treatment of pragmatic disorder in children. Child Language Teaching and Therapy 10: 1–22.

Levitt L, Muir J (1983) Which three-year-olds need speech therapy? Use of Levitt–Muir Screening Test. Health Visitor 56: 454–56.

Lewis BA (1990) Familial phonological disorders: four pedigrees. Journal of Speech and Hearing Disorders 55: 160–70.

Lewis BA, Thompson LA (1992) A study of developmental speech and language disorders in twins. Journal of Speech and Hearing Research 35: 1086–94.

Lewis M (1977) Social behaviour and language acquisition. In Lewis M, Rosenbloom LA (Eds) Interaction, Communication and the Development of Language. New York: John Wiley.

Lewis M, Bendersky M (1989) Cognitive and motor differences among low birthweight infants: Impact of intraventricular haemorrhage, medical risk and social class. Pediatrics 83: 187–92.

Lewis M, Freedle R (1973) Mother–infant dyad: The cradle of meaning. In Pliner P, Kramer L, Alloway T (Eds) Communication and Affect: Language and Thought. New York: Academic Press.

Liberman AM, Cooper FS, Shankweiler DP, Studdert-Kennedy M (1967) Perception of the speech code. Psychology Review 74: 431–61.

Lieven EVM (1978) Conversations between mothers and young children: Individual differences and their possible implication for the study of language learning. In Waterson N, Snow C (Eds) Development of Communication. New York: John Wiley.

Lieven EVM (1982) Context, process and progress in young children's speech. In Beveridge M (Ed.) Children Thinking Through Language. London: Edward Arnold.

Lieven E, Pine J, Dresner Barnes H (1992) Individual differences in early vocabulary development: redefining the referential–expressive distinction. Journal of Child Language 19: 287–310.

Lindsay G (Ed.) (1984) Screening for Children with Special Needs. London: Croom Helm.

Lister Brook S, Bowler D (1992) Autism by another name? Semantic and pragmatic impairments in children. Journal of Autism and Developmental Disorders 22: 61–81.

Lloyd P (1982) Talking to some purpose. In Beveridge M (Ed.) Children Thinking Through Language. London: Edward Arnold.

Locke A (1985) Living Language. Windsor: NFER-Nelson.

Locke A (1989) Screening and intervention with children with speech and language difficulties in mainstream schools. In Mogford K, Sadler J (Eds) Child Language Disability. Implications in an Educational Setting. Avon: Multilingual Matters.

Locke JL (1980) The inference of speech perception in the phonologically disordered child. Parts 1 and 2. Journal of Speech and Hearing Disorders 45: 431–68.

Locke JL (1983) Phonological Acquisition and Change. New York: Academic Press.

Locke JL (1986) The linguistic significance of language. In Lindblom B, Zetterstrom R (Eds) Precursors of Early Speech. Werner–Gren International Symposium, Series, 44. Basingstoke: MacMillan Press. (New York: Stockton Press.)

Locke JL (1994) Gradual emergence of developmental language disorders. Journal of Speech and Hearing Research 37: 608–16

Long SH, Hand L (1996) Acquisition of lexical semantic fields: an evaluation of the PRISM-L. Child Language, Teaching and Therapy 12: 206–30.

Lonigan CJ, Fischel JE, Whitehurst GJ, Arnold DS, Valdez-Menchaca MC (1992) The role of otitis media in the development of expressive language delay. Developmental Psychology 28: 430–40.

Ludlow C, Cooper JA (Eds) (1983) Genetic Aspects of Speech and Language Disorders. New York: Academic Press.

Lund NJ (1986) Family events and relationships. Seminars in speech and language, Vol. 4. New York: Thieme Medical.

Lund NJ, Duchan J (1983, 1987) Assessing Children's Language in Naturalistic Contexts, (First and Second Edn.) Englewood Cliffs, NJ: Prentice Hall.

Luria AR (1970) Traumatic Aphasia. The Hague: Mouton.

Luria AR (1973) The Working Brain. London: Allen Lane, The Penguin Press.

Mac Keith R, Rutter M (1972) A note on the prevalence of speech and language disorders. In Rutter M, Martin JAM (Eds) The Child with Delayed Speech. Clinics in Developmental Medicine, 43. London: SIMP with Heineman Medical.

MacNeilage PF (1970) Motor control and serial ordering of speech. Psychological Review 75: 182–96

Marge M (1972) The general problem of language disabilities in children. In Irwin JV, Marge M (Eds) The Principles of Childhood Language Disabilities. New York: Appleton-Century-Crofts.

Marge M (1984) The prevention of communication disorders. ASHA 26: 29–34.

Marlaire CL, Maynard DW (1990) Standardised testing as an interactional phenomenon. Sociology of Education 63: 83–101.

Marshall JC (1983) Preface to Aphasiology, Lecours AH, L'Hermitte F, Bryans B (Eds). London: Baillière Tindall.

Marshall J, Newcombe F (1973) Patterns of paralexia: a psycholinguistic approach. Journal of Psycholinguistic Research 2: 175–99.

Marshman A, Miller C (1994) Integration of a pupil from a language unit into the host school. Child Language Teaching and Therapy 10: 299–312.

Marslen-Wilson WD, Tyler LK (1980) The temporal structure of spoken language: understanding. Cognition 8: 1–71.

Martin D, Reilly O (1995) Global language delay: analysis of a severe central auditory processing deficit. In Perkins M, Howard S (Eds.) Case Studies in Clinical Linguistics. London: Whurr.

McCarthy R, Warrington E (1990) Cognitve neuropsycholgy: a clinical introduction. London: Academic Press.

McCartney E (1993) The assessment of expressive language. In Beech J, Harding L (with Hilton-Jones D) Assessment in Speech and Language Therapy. London: Routledge.

McCauley R (Ed.) (1988) Language, Speech and Reading Disorders in Children: Neuropsychological Studies of RE Stark and P Tallal. Boston, MA: College-Hill.

McCauley R, Swisher L (1984) Use and misuse of norm-referenced tests in clinical assessment: A hypothetical case. Journal of Speech and Hearing Disorders 49: 338–48.

McGinnis M (1963) Aphasic Children. Washington DC: Alexander Graham Bell Association for the Deaf Inc.

McGregor KK, Leonard LB (1995) Intervention for word-finding deficits in children. In Fey M, Windsor J, Warren SF (Eds) Language Intervention: Preschool Through the Elementary Years. Baltimore, MD: Paul Brookes.

McLaughlin CS, Gullow DF (1984) Comparison of three formal methods of preschool language assessment. Language, Speech and Hearing Services in Schools 15: 145–53.

McTear M (1985) Pragmatic disorders: a case study of conversational disability. British Journal of Disorders of Communication 20: 129–41.

McTear M, Conti-Ramsden G (1992) Pragmatic disability in children. London: Whurr.

McWhinney B, Bates E (1989) The crosslinguistic study of language processing. Cambridge: Cambridge University Press.

Menyuk P, Looney PL (1972) Relationships among components of the grammar in language disorders. Journal of Speech and Hearing Research 15: 395–406.

Menyuk P, Liebergott J, Schultz M (1986) Predicting phonological development. In Lindblom B, Zetterstrom R (Eds) Precursors of Early Speech. Werner–Gren, International Symposium Series 44. Basingstoke: Macmillan Press. (New York: Stockton Press.)

Menyuk P, Liebergott J, Schultz M, Chesnick M, Ferrier L (1991) Patterns of early lexical and cognitive development in premature and full-term infants. Journal of Speech and Hearing Research 34: 88–94.

Miller GA (1967) The magical number of 7 plus or minus 2. The Psychology of Communication. Harmondsworth: Penguin.

Miller JF (1981) Assessing Language Production in Children. London: Edward Arnold.

Miller JF (1987) A grammatical characterisation of language disorder. In Proceedings of First International Symposium. Specific Speech and Language Disorders in Children, University of Reading. London: AFASIC.

Miller JF (1991a) Research on child language disorders in children : a progress report. In Miller JF (Ed.) Research in Child Language Disorders: A Decade of Progress. Austin, TX: Pro-ed.

Miller JF (1991b) Quantifying productive language disorders. In Miller JF (Ed.) Research in Child Language Disorders: A Decade of Progress. Austin, TX: Pro-ed.

Miller L (1984) Problem solving and language remediation. In Wallach GP, Butler KG (Eds) Language Learning Disabilities in School Aged Children. Baltimore, MD: Williams and Wilkins.

Moray N (1972) Listening and Attention. Harmondsworth: Penguin Books.

Morgan-Barry, R. (1988) Language use versus phonology versus prosody: A spin-off effect. Unpublished Paper.

Morley ME (1960) Developmental receptive–expressive dysphasia. Speech and Pathology Therapy 3: 64–76.

Morley ME (1972) Development and Disorders of Speech in Childhood, (Third Edn). Edinburgh: Churchill Livingstone.

Morley ME (1973) Receptive/expressive developmental aphasia. British Journal of Disorders of Communication. 8: 47–53.

Morton J (1978) Facilitation in word recognition: experiments causing change in the logogen model. In Koiers PA, Wrolstad ME, Bouma H (Eds) Proceedings of the Conference on the Processing of Visible Language. New York: Plenum.

Muir A (1992) Workshops work! Bulletin of the College of Speech and Language Therapists, July.

Muller DJ, Munro S, Code C (1981) Language Assessment for Remediation. London: Croom Helm.

Muma JR (1978) Language Handbook. Concepts, Assessment, Intervention. Englewood Cliffs, New Jersey: Prentice Hall.

Muma JR (1983) Speech–language pathology: Emerging clinical expertise in language. In Gallagher TM, Prutting CA (Eds) Pragmatic Assessment and Intervention in Language. San Diego, CA: College Hill Press.

Murdoch B (1990) Acquired Speech and Language Disorders in Children. London: Chapman and Hall.

Mysak ED (1976) Pathologies of Speech Systems. Baltimore, MD: Williams and Wilkins.

Netsell R (1986) A Neurobiologic View of Speech Production and the Dysarthrias. San Diego, CA: College Hill Press.

Newman S (1996) Working on both sides of the fence: the effect of a dual qualification on collaborative working practice. Child Language Teaching and Therapy 11: 39–47.

Nippold M (1992) The nature of normal and disordered word finding in children and adolescents. Topics in Language Disorders 13: 1–14.

Norris J, Hoffman P (1993) Whole language intervention for school-age children. San Diego, CA: Singular Publishing Group.

Nye C, Foster S, Seaman D (1987) Effectiveness of intervention with the language/learning disabled. Journal of Speech and Hearing Disorders 52: 348–57.

Oller DK (1980) The emergence of the sounds of speech in infancy. In Yeni-KomshianGH, Kavanagh JF, Ferguson CA (Eds) Child Phonology: Volume I. Production, New York: Academic Press.

Olswang LB, Bain BA (1996) Assessment information for predicting upcoming change in language production. Journal of Speech and Hearing Research 39: 414–23.

Omura T (1991) A longitudinal study of the relationship between early language development and play development. Journal of Child Language 18: 273–94.

Owrid HL (1970) Hearing impairment and verbal attainment in primary school children. Educational Research 12: 209–14.

Panagos JM, Bobkoff K (1984) Beliefs about developmental apraxia of speech. Australian Journal of Human Communication Disorders 12: 40–53.

Panagos JM, Quine ME, Klich RJ (1979) Syntactic and phonological influences on children's articulation. Journal of Speech and Hearing Research 22: 829–40.

Panagos JM, Bobkoff K, Scott CM (1986) Discourse analysis of language intervention. Child Language and Teaching Therapy 2: 211–29.

Panagos JM, Bobkoff-Katz K, Kovarsky D, Prelock PA (1988) The non-verbal component of clinical lessons. Child Language Teaching and Therapy 4: 228–96.

Paradise JL (1981) Otitis media in early life. How hazardous to development? A critical review of the evidence. Pediatrics 68: 869–73.

Paul R (1992) Language and speech disorders. In Hooper S, Hynd GW, Mattison RE (Eds) Developmental Disorders: Diagnostic Criteria and Clinical Assessment. Hillsdale, NJ: Lawrence Erlbaum.

Paul R (1995) Language Disorders: From Infancy Through Adolescence. St Louis, MD: Mosby Year Book.

Paul R, Cohen DJ (1984) Outcomes of severe disorders of language acquisition. Journal of Autism and Developmental Disorders 14: 405–21.

Pembrey M (1992) Genetics and language disorder. In Fletcher P, Hall D (Eds) Specific Speech and Language Disorders in Children. London: Whurr.

Plante E (1991) MRI findings in the parents and siblings of specific language-impaired boys. Brain and Language 41: 67–80.

Plante E, Swisher L, Vance R, Rapcsak S (1991) MRI findings in boys with specific language impairment. Brain and Language 41: 52–66.

Prescott P, De Caspar AJ (1990) Human perception of speech and nonspeech is functionally lateralised at birth. Manuscript submitted for publication cited in Flavell, Miller and Miller (1993).

Proctor A (1982) Use of linguistic input in clinical assessment. Miniseminar presented at the Annual Convention of American Speech Language and Hearing Association, Toronto.

Prutting CA, Gallagher TM, Mulac A (1975) The expressive portion of the NWSST compared to a spontaneous language sample. Journal of Speech and Hearing Disorders 40: 40–9.

Prutting CA, Kirchner DM (1983) Applied pragmatics. In Gallagher TM, Prutting CA (Eds) Pragmatic Assessment and Intervention Issues in Language. San Diego, CA: College Hill Press.

Randall D, Reynell J, Curwen M (1974) A study of language development in a sample of three-year-old children. British Journal of Disorders of Communication 9: 3–16.

Rapin I, Allen DA (1983) Developmental language disorders: nosological considerations. In Kirk U (Ed.) Neuropsychology of Language, Reading and Spelling. New York: Academic Press.

Rapin I, Allen DA (1987) Developmental dysphasia and autism in preschool children. In Proceedings of First International Symposium. Specific Speech and Language Disorders in Children, University of Reading. London: AFASIC.

Rees N (1973) Auditory processing factors in language disorders: the view from Procrustes' bed. Journal of Speech and Hearing Disorders 38: 304–15.

Rescorla L (1984) Language delay in two-year-olds. Paper presented at Fourth International Symposium of Infant Studies, New York.

Rescorla L (1989) The Language Development Survey: a screening tool for delayed language in toddlers. Journal of Speech and Hearing Research 54: 587–99.

Rescorla L (1993) Use of parental report in the identification of communicatively delayed toddlers. Seminars in Speech and Language 14: 264–77.

Rescorla L, Hadicke-Wiley M, Escarce E (1993) Epidemiological investigation of expressive language delay at age two. First Language 13: 5–22.

Reynell JK (1969) A developmental approach to language disorders. British Journal of Disorders of Communication 4: 38–40.

Rice ML (1983) Contemporary accounts of the cognition/language relationship. Implications for speech–language clinicians. Journal of Speech and Hearing Disorders 48: 347–59.

Ripich DN, Panagos JM (1985) Accessing children's knowledge of sociolinguistic rules for speech therapy lessons. Journal of Speech and Hearing Disorders 50: 346–55.

Ripley K (1987) Counselling children with specific speech and language disorders. Proceedings of First International Symposium Specific Speech and Language Disorders in Children, University of Reading. London: AFASIC.

Roberts JE, Schuele CM (1991) Otitis media and later academic performance: the linkage and implications for intervention. Topics in Language Disorders 11: 43–62.

Roberts JE, Burchinal MR, Davis BP, Collier AM, Henderson FW (1991) Otitis media in early childhood and later language. Journal of Speech and Hearing Research 34: 1158–68.

Robinson RJ (1987) The causes of language disorder. Proceedings of first International Symposium Specific Speech and Language Disorders in Children, University of Reading. London: AFASIC.

Robinson RJ (1991) Brain imaging and language. In Fletcher P, Hall D (Eds) Specific Speech and Language Disorders in Children. London: Whurr.

Rosenbek J (1974) Treatment of developmental apraxia of speech: A case study. Language, Speech and Hearing Services in Schools 5: 13–22.

Rutter M (Ed.) (1984) Issues and prospects in developmental neuropsychiatry. In Developmental Neuropsychiatry. Edinburgh: Churchill Livingstone.

Rutter M (1987) Developmental language disorders: Some thoughts on causes and correlates. Proceedings of First International Symposium on Specific Speech and Language Disorders in Children, University of Reading. London: AFASIC.

Rutter M, Lord C (1987) Language disorder associated with psychiatric disturbance. In Yule W, Rutter M (Eds) Language Development and Disorders. Oxford: SIMP, Blackwell Scientific and Lippincott.

Rutter M, Bartak L, Newman S (1971) Autism: A central disorder of cognition and language? In Rutter M (Ed.) Infantile Autism. Concepts, Characteristics and Treatment. Edinburgh: Churchill Livingstone.

Sarno M (1993) Aphasia rehabilitation: psychosocial and ethical considerations. Aphasiology 7: 321–34.

Savic S (1980) How Twins Learn to Talk. London: Academic Press.

Schery TK (1985) Correlates of language development in language-disordered children. Journal of Speech and Hearing Disorders 50: 73–83.

Shaffer LH (1992) Motor programming and control. In Stelmach G, Requin J (Eds) Tutorials in Motor Behaviour. North Holland: Elsevier Science.

Shallice T (1984) More functionally isolable systems but fewer 'modules'? Cognition 17: 243–52.

Shore CM (1995) Individual differences in language development. Thousand Oaks, CA: Sage Publications.

Shriberg LD, Smith AJ (1983) Phonological correlates of middle ear involvement in speech-delayed children: a methodological note. Journal of Speech and Hearing Research 26: 293–97.

Siegel GM, Katsuki J, Potechin G (1985) Response to contemporary accounts of the cognition/language relationship. Journal of Speech and Hearing Disorders 50: 281–317.

Silva PA (1980) The prevalence, stability and significance of developmental language delay in preschool children. Developmental Medicine and Child Neurology 22: 768–77.

Silva PA, Ferguson D (1980) Some factors contributing to language development in three-year-old children. British Journal of Disorders of Communication 15: 200–14.

Silva PA, McGee RO, Williams SM (1983) Developmental language delay from three to seven years and its significance for low intelligence and reading difficulties at age seven. Developmental Medicine and Child Neurology 25: 783–93.

Sinclair de Zwart H (1969) Developmental psycholinguistics. In Elkind D, Flavell J (Eds) Studies in Cognitive Development. Oxford: Oxford University Press.

Skuse D (1991) The relationship between physical deprivation, physical growth and the impaired development of language. In Fletcher P, Hall D (Eds) Specific Speech and Language Disorders in Children. London: Whurr.

Smedley M (1989) Semantic–pragmatic language disorder: a description with some practical suggestions for teachers. Child Language, Teaching and Therapy 5: 174–90.

Smith BR, Leinonen E (1992) Clinical Pragmatics. London: Chapman and Hall.

Smith, N, Tsimpli I (1995) The Mind of a Savant: Language Learning and Modularity. Oxford: Blackwell Science.

Snow CE (1972) Mothers' speech to children learning language. Child Development 13: 549–65.

Snow CE, Ferguson CA (Eds) (1977) Talking to Children: Language Input and Acquisition. Cambridge: Cambridge University Press.

Snowling M (Ed.) (1985a) Postscript: Some consistencies and contradictions: directions for future research. In Children's Written Language Difficulties. Windsor: NFER-Nelson.

Snowling M (1985b) Dyslexia care–the therapist's crucial role. Speech Therapy in Practice 13: 21–2.

Snowling M (1987) Dyslexia: A Cognitive Developmental Perspective. Oxford: Blackwell Science.

Snyder L (1982) Defining language–disordered children: Disordered or just 'Low Verbal' normal? Proceedings of Third Symposium on Research in Child Language Disorders, Madison, WI.

Snyder L, Godley D (1992) Assessment of word-finding disorders in children and adolescents. Topics in Language Disorders 13: 15–32.

Snyder-McClean L, McClean JE (1987) Effectiveness of early intervention for children with language and communicative disorders. In Guralnick MJ, Bennett FC (Eds) The Effectiveness of Early Intervention for At-risk and Handicapped Children. New York: Academic Press.

Sommers RK (1991) Approaches to the prediction of language abilities in a sample of children having language delays. Journal of Speech and Hearing Research 34: 317–24.

Sonksen P (1979) The neurodevelopmental and paediatric findings associated with significant disabilities of language development. Unpublished MD Thesis, University of London.

Sparks SN (1989) Assessment and intervention with at-risk infants and toddlers: guidelines for speech–language pathologists. Topics in Language Disorders 10: 43–56.

Spencer A (1986) Towards a theory of phonological development. Lingua 68: 3–38.

Sperber D, Wilson D (1987) Relevance: Communication and Cognition. Oxford: Blackwell Science.

Springer SP, Deutsch G (1989) Left Brain, Right Brain, (Third Edn). San Francisco, CA: W.H. Freeman.

Stackhouse J (1982) An investigation of reading and spelling performance in speech disordered children. British Journal of Disorders of Communication 17: 53–60.

Stackhouse J (1984) Phonological therapy–a case and some thoughts. Bulletin of the College of Speech Therapists, January.

Stackhouse J (1985) Segmentation, speech and spelling difficulties. In Snowling M (Ed.) Children's Written Language Difficulties. Windsor: NFER-Nelson.

Stackhouse J (1992) Developmental verbal dyspraxia. I: A review and critique. European Journal of Disorders of Communication 27: 19–34.

Stackhouse J (1993) Phonological disorder and lexical development: two case studies. Child Language Teaching and Therapy 9: 230–41.

Stackhouse J, Wells B (1993) Psycholinguistic assessment of speech disorders. European Journal of Disorders of Communication 28: 331–47.

Stark RE (1981) Stages of speech development in the first year of life. In Yeni-Komshian GH, Kavanagh JF, Ferguson CA (Eds) Child Phonology, Vol. I. Production. New York: Academic Press.

Stark RE, Tallal P (1981) Selection of children with specific language impairment. Journal of Speech and Hearing Disorders 46: 114–22.

Stark RE, Mellits E, Tallal P (1983) Behavioral attributes of speech and language disorders. In Ludlow CL, Cooper JA (Eds) Genetic Aspects of Speech and Language Disorders. New York: Academic Press.

Stark RE, Tallal P, Mellits E (1985) Expressive language and perceptual motor abilities in language-impaired children. Human Communication (Canada) 9: 23–8.

Stelmach GE (1982) Information-processing framework for understanding human motor behavior. In Scott Kelso J (Ed.) Human Motor Behaviour. Hillsdale, NJ: Lawrence Erlbaum.

Stelmach GE, Kelso JAS, Wallace SA (1975) Preselection in short term motor memory. Journal of Experimental Psychology 1: 745–55.

Stemberger JP (1992) A connectionist view of child phonology: Phonological processing without phonological processes. In Ferguson C, Menn L, Stoel-Gammon C (Eds) Phonological Development: Models, Research, Implications. Timonium: York Press.

Stevenson J, Richman N (1976) The prevalence of language delay in a population of three-year-old children and its association with general retardation. Developmental Medicine and Child Neurology 18: 431–41.

Stevenson P, Bax M, Stevenson J (1982) The evaluation of home-based speech therapy for language delayed preschool children in an inner city area. British Journal of Disorders of Communication 17: 141–48.

Stoel-Gammon C, Herrington P (1990) Vowel systems of normally-developing and phonologically-disordered children. Clinical Linguistics and Phonetics 4: 145–60.

Stone E (1992) A follow-up study of ex-pupils from a speech and language therapy unit. Child Language Teaching and Therapy 8: 285–313.

Stothard SE, Snowling MJ, Bishop DVM, Chipchase BB, Kaplan C (1996) Language impaired preschoolers: a follow-up into adolescence (in press).

Strominger AZ, Bashir AS (1977) A nine year follow-up of language-delayed children. Paper presented at Annual Convention of the American Speech Language and Hearing Association, Chicago, L.

Tallal P (1987) The neuropsychology of developmental language disorders. Proceedings of First International Symposium. Specific Speech and Language Disorders in Children, University of Reading. London: AFASIC.

Tallal P, Piercy M (1978) Defects of auditory perception in children with developmental dysphasia. In Wyke M (Ed.) Developmental Dysphasia. London: Academic Press.

Tallal P, Ross R, Curtiss S (1989) Familial aggregation in specific language impairment. Journal of Speech and Hearing Disorders 54: 167–73.

Tallal P, Townsend J, Curtiss S, Wulfeck B (1991) Phenotypic profiles of language-impaired children based on genetic/family history. Brain and Language 41: 81–95.

Teele DW, Klein JO, Rosner BA, The Greater Boston Otitis Media Study Group (1984) Otitis media with effusion during the first three years of life, and development of language. Pediatrics 74: 282–87.

Tempest B, Parkinson E (1993) A case study of a child with severe dyspraxia and reading difficulties. Child Language Teaching and Therapy 9: 242–50.

Tew B (1979) The 'Cocktail Party Syndrome' in children with hydrocephalus and spina bifida. British Journal of Disorders of Communication 14: 89–101.

Thal D, Bates E (1988) Language and gesture in late talkers. Journal of Speech and Hearing Research 31: 115–23.

Thal D, Tobias S, Morrison D (1991) Language and gesture in late talkers: a 1-year follow-up. Journal of Speech and Hearing Research 34: 604–12.

Thomas ME (1969) Assessment and treatment of receptive and executive aphasia in identical twin boys. British Journal of Disorders of Communication 4: 57–63.

Tomblin JB (1989) Familial concentration of developmental language impairment. Journal of Speech and Hearing Disorders 54: 287–95.

Tomblin JB, Buckwalter PR (1994) Studies of genetics in specific language impairment. In Watkins RV, Rice ML (Eds) Specific Language Impairments in Children. Baltimore, MD: Paul Brookes.

Trevarthen C, Marwick H (1986) Signs of motivation for speech in infants and the nature of a mother's support for development of language. In Lindblom B, Zetterstrom R (Eds) Precursors of Early Speech. Werner–Gren International Symposium Series 44. Basingstoke: Macmillan Press. (New York: Stockton Press.)

Trevarthen C, Murray L, Hubley P (1981) Psychology of infants. In Davis J, Dobbing J (Eds) Scientific Foundations of Paediatrics, 2nd Edn. London: William Heineman Medical.

Tuomi SK, Ivanoff P (1977) Incidence of speech and hearing disorders among kindergarten and Grade one children. Special Education in Canada 51: 5–8.

Turton LJ (1983) Curriculum concepts for language treatment of children. In Winitz H (Ed.) Treating Language Disorders. Baltimore, MD: Baltimore University Park Press.

United States of America Public Law (1975) Education for All Handicapped Children Act, PL 94–142.

United States of America Public Law (1986) Education of the Handicapped Act. Amendment Title I Handicapped Infants and Toddlers, PL 99–457.

Vance M (1991) Educational and therapeutic approaches used with a child presenting with acquired aphasia with convulsive disorder (Landau–Kleffner syndrome). Child Language Teaching and Therapy 7: 41–60.

Van Der Gaag A, Davies P (1994) Following the dolphins: an ethnographic study of speech and language therapy with people with learning difficulties. European

Journal of Disorders of Communication 29: 203–23.

Van Der Lely HJK (1990) Sentence comprehension processes in specifically language-impaired children. Unpublished PhD thesis: University of London.

Van Der Lely H (1993) Specific language impairment in children: research findings and their therapeutic implications. European Journal of Disorders of Communication 28: 247–61.

Van Der Lely HJK (1994) Canonical linking rules:forward versus reverse linking in normally developing and specifically language impaired children. Cognition 51: 29–72.

Van Der Lely HJK (1996) Empirical evidence for the modularity of language from grammatical SLI children. Proceedings from the Boston University Conference on Language Development, 20. Boston, MA: Cascadilla Press (forthcoming).

Van Der Lely HJK, Dewart H (1986) Sentence comprehension strategies in specifically language-impaired children. British Journal of Disorders of Communication 21: 291–306.

Van Der Lely HJK, Harris M (1990) Comprehension of reversible passives in specifically language-impaired children. Journal of Speech and Hearing Disorders 55: 101–17.

Van Der Lely HJK, Stollwerck L (1996) A grammatical specific language impairment in children: An autosomal dominant inheritance? Brain and Language 52: 1–21.

Van Der Stelt JM, Koopmans Van Beinum FJ (1986) The onset of babbling related to gross motor development. In Lindblom B, Zetterstrom R (Eds) Precursors of Early Speech. Werner–Gren International Symposium Series 44. Basingstoke: Macmillan Press. (New York: Stockton Press.)

Van Kleeck A (1981) Children's development of metalinguistic skills. Communicative Disorders; Vol 6. 9, An Audio Journal for Continuing Education. New York: Grune and Stratton.

Ventry I (1980) Effects of hearing loss. Fact or fiction? Journal of Speech and Hearing Disorders 45: 143–56.

Walton JN, Ellis E, Court SDM (1962) Clumsy children: developmental apraxia and agnosia. Brain 85: 603–12.

Ward S (1984) Detecting abnormal auditory behaviours in infancy: the relationship between such behaviours and linguistic development. British Journal of Disorders of Communication 19: 237–51.

Ward S (1996) Seminar presented at the Centre for Audiology, Education of the Deaf and Speech Pathology University of Manchester, April 1996.

Ward S, Kellett B (1982) Language disorder resolved? British Journal of Disorders of Communication 17: 32–52.

Ward S, McCartney E (1978) Congenital auditory imperception. A follow-up study. British Journal of Disorders of Communication 13: 1–6.

Warner JAW (1987) Cerebral palsy: a chance to influence the environment. Speech Therapy in Practice 2: 5–7.

Warner J, Byers-Brown B, McCartney E (1984) Speech Therapy. A Clinical Companion. Manchester: Manchester University Press.

Watkins RV, Rice ML (Eds) (1994) Specific language impairments in children. Baltimore, MD: Paul Brookes.

Wedell K (1980) Early intervention. In Knight RN, Bakker DJ (Eds) Early Identification and Treatment of Hyperactive Children. Baltimore, MD: University Park Press.

Weeks ST (1974) The Slow Speech Development of a Bright Child. Lexington, MA: Lexington Books

Weiner P, Hoock W (1973) The standardisation of tests: criteria and criticisms.

Journal of Speech and Hearing Research 16: 616–26.

Weiss CE, Gordon ME, Lillywhite HS (1987) Clinical Management of Articulatory and Phonological Disorders (Second Edn) Baltimore, MD: Williams and Wilkins.

Weistuch L, Byers Brown B (1987) Motherese as therapy: programme and its dissemination. Child Language Teaching and Therapy 3: 57–72.

Wells B (1994) Junction in developmental speech disorder: a case study. Journal of Clinical Linguistics and Phonetics 8: 1–25.

Wells B, Local J (1993) The sense of an ending, a case of prosodic delay. Clinical Linguistics and Phonetics 7: 59–73.

Wells G (1985) Language Development in the Preschool Years. Cambridge: Cambridge University Press.

Westby CE (1984) Development of narrative language abilities. In Wallach GP, Butler KG (Eds) Language Learning Disabilities in School-age Children. Baltimore, MD: Williams and Wilkins.

Wetherby A, Cain D, Yonelas A, Walker V (1986) Intentional communication in the emerging language of normal infants. Mini-seminar presentation at Annual Convention of American Speech, Language and Hearing Association, Detroit, MI.

Whitehurst GJ, Fischel JE (1994) Practitioner review: Early developmental language delay: What, if anything, should the clinician do about it? Journal of Child Psychology and Psychiatry 35: 613–48.

Whitehurst GJ, Falco FL, Lonigen CJ, Fischel JE, De Baryshe BD, Valdez-Menchaca MC, Caulfield M (1988) Accelerating language development through picture book reading. Developmental Psychology 24: 690–99.

Whitehurst GJ, Arnold DS, Smith M, Fischel JE, Lonigan CJ, Valdez-Menchaca MC (1991) Family history in developmental expressive language delay. Journal of Speech and Hearing Research 34: 1150–57.

Wiig E (1987) Strategic language use in adolescents with learning disabilities: Assessment and education. Proceedings of First International Symposium Specific Speech and Language Disorders in Children, University of Reading. London: AFASIC.

Wiig E (1995) Assessments of adolescent language. Seminars in Speech and Language 16(1): 14–31.

Wiig E, Semel E. (1984) Language Assessment and Intervention for the Learning Disabled. Columbus, OH: Charles E Merrill.

Wiig E, Becker-Caplan L (1984) Linguistic retrieval strategies and word-finding difficulties among children with language disabilities. Topics in Language Disorders 4: 1–18.

Williams A (1996) Cracking the code. Bulletin of the Royal College of Speech and Language Therapists, April, 9–10.

Williams N, Chiat S (1993) Processing deficits in children with phonological disorder and delay. Clinical Linguistics and Phonetics 7: 145–57.

Williams P, Corrin J (1995) The Nuffield Dyspraxia Programme update. Poster Presentation at the Golden Jubilee Conference of the Royal College of Speech Therapists, York.

Williams R, Ingham R, Rosenthal J (1981) A further analysis for developmental apraxia of speech in children with defective articulation. Journal of Speech and Hearing Research 24: 496–505.

Wilson BC (1979) Precursors of learning disability. Paper presented at International Neuropsychological Society, Noordurjerhool, The Netherlands.

Wilson BC (1981) Longitudinal studies of preschool disordered children. Paper presented at The Orton Society Conference, New York.

Wilson BC, Risucci DA (1986) A model for clinical quantitative classification: Generation 1. Application to language-disordered preschool children. Brain and Language 27: 281–309.

Winitz H (1969) Articulatory Acquisition and Behavior. New York: Appleton-Century-Crofts.

Wirz S (1993) Historical considerations in assessment. In Beech J, Harding L, Hilton-Jones D (Eds) Assessment in Speech and Language Therapy. London: Routledge.

Wolff PH, Gunnoe C, Cohen C (1985) Neuromotor maturation and psychological performance: a developmental study. Developmental Medicine and Child Neurology 27: 344–54.

Wolfus B, Moscovitch M, Kinsbourne M (1980) Subgroups of developmental language impairment. Brain and Language 10: 152–71.

Wolf-Schein EG, Sudhalter V, Cohen IL, Fisch GS, Hanson D, Pfadt AG, Hagerman R, Jenkins EC, Brown WT (1987) Speech–language and the Fragile X syndrome. ASHA, July, 35–38.

Woods BT, Carey S (1979) Language deficits after apparent recovery from childhood aphasia. Annals of Neurology 6: 405–9.

World Health Organisation (1980) Early Detection of Handicap in Children. Geneva: WHO.

Worster-Drought C, Allen IM (1930) Congenital auditory imperception. Journal of Neurology and Psychopathology 10: 193–236.

Wright J (1996) Teachers and therapists : the evolution of a partnership. Child Language Teaching and Therapy 12: 3–16.

Wright NE, Thistlethwaite D, Elton RA, Wilkinson EM, Forfar JO (1983) The speech and language development of low birthweight infants. British Journal of Disorders of Communication 18: 187–96.

Wyke M (Ed.) (1978) Developmental Dysphasia. London: Academic Press.

Yoss KA, Darley FL (1974a) Developmental apraxia of speech in children with defective articulation. Journal of Speech and Hearing Research 17: 399–416.

Yoss KA, Darley FL (1974b) Therapy in developmental apraxia of speech. Language, Speech and Hearing Services in Schools 5: 23–31.

Principal tests cited in text

Anthony A, Bogle D, Ingram TTS, McIsaac M (1971) Edinburgh Articulation Test. Edinburgh: Livingstone.

Arthur G (1952) Leiter International Performance Scale (adaptation). Washington DC: Psychological Services Center.

Bayley N (1969) Bayley Scales of Infant Development. New York: The Psychological Corporation.

Bishop DVM (1983) Test for Reception of Grammar. Available from the author, Department of Psychology, University of Manchester.

Capute AJ, Palmer FB, Shapiro BK. Wachtel RC, Schmidt S, Ross A (1986) Clinical and Auditory Milestone Scale. Prediction of cognition in infancy. Developmental Medicine and Child Neurology 28: 762–71.

Carrow Wolfolk E (1973, revised 1985) Test for Auditory Comprehension of Language Windsor: NFER.

Carrow Wolfolk E (1974) Carrow Elicited Language Inventory. Windsor: NFER.

Dewart H, Summers S (1988) Pragmatic and Early Communication Profile. Windsor: NFER.

Doll EA (1965) Vineland Maturity Scale. Minneapolis, MN: American Guidance Service.

Frankenburg WK, Fandal AW, Sciarelto W, Burgess D (1981) The Newly Abbreviated and Revised Denver Developmental Screening Test. Journal of Pediatrics 99: 995–99.

French JL (1964) Pictorial Test of Intelligence. New York: Houghton Mifflin.

German D (1986/1989) National College of Education Test of Word Finding Skills (TWF) Allen, TX: DLM Teaching Resources.

German DJ (1989) National College of Education Test of Word Finding. Allen, TX: DLM Teaching Resources.

Goldman R, Fristoe N, Woodcock RW (1972) Goldman–Fristoe–Woodcock Test of Auditory Discrimination. Circle Pines, Minneapolis, MN: American Guidance Service.

Grunwell P (1982) Phonological Assessment of Children's Speech. Windsor: NFER.

Gutfreund M, Harrison M, Wells G (1989) Bristol Language Development Scales. Windsor: NFER.

Hedrick DL, Prather EM, Tobin AE (1975) Sequenced Inventory of Communication Development. Seattle, WA: Seattle University Press.

Hiskey MS (1966) Hiskey–Nebraska Test of Learning Aptitude. Lincoln, NE: Union College Press.

Kirk SA, McCarthy JJ, Kirk WD (1968) Illinois Test of Psycholinguistic Abilities. Urbana, IL: University of Illinois Press.

Knowles W, Masidlover M (1987) The Derbyshire Language Scheme (revised) Educational Psychology Service, Derbyshire County Council.

Lee L (1969) North Western Syntax Screening Test. Evanston, IL: North Western University Press.

McCarthy D (1974) McCarthy Scales of Children's Abilities. New York: The Psychological Corporation.

Meecham N (1958) Verbal Language Development Scale, Revised, 1971. Circle Pines, Minneapolis, MN: American Guidance Service.

Morgan-Barry R (1988) Auditory Discrimination and Attention Test. Windsor: NFER.

PORCH (1972) Porch Index of Communicative Abilities (PICA), Palo Alto: Consulting Psychologists Press.

Renfrew CE (1972a) Auditory Discrimination Test. Obtainable from the author, 2a North Place, Old Headington, Oxford OX3 9HX.

Renfrew CE (1972b) The Bus Story. Bicester: Winslow Press.

Renfrew CE (1988) Action Picture Test (revised). Bicester: Winslow Press.

Reynell J (1977; 1985 revised edn) Reynell Language Development Scales. Windsor: NFER.

Semel EM, Wiig E, Secord W (1987) Clinical Evaluation of Language Fundamentals-Revised. San Antonio, TX: Psychological Corporation.

Shulman BB (1985) Test of Pragmatic Skills. Tucson, AZ: Communication Skill Builders.

Templin M (1957) Certain Language Skills in Children. Minneapolis, MN: University of Minnesota Press.

Wechsler D (1967) Wechsler Pre-school and Primary Scale of Intelligence (WIPPSI). New York: Process Analysis. Baltimore, MD: University Park Press.

Wepman J (1973) Auditory Discrimination Test. Chicago, IL: Language Research Association.

Wheldall K, Mittler P, Hobsbaum A, (1987) Sentence Comprehension Test. Windsor: NFER–Nelson.

Wiig E, Secord W (1989) Test of Language Competence-expanded. San Antonio, TX: Psychological Corporation.

Wiig E, Secord W (1992) Test of Word Knowledge. San Antonio, TX: Psychological Corporation.

Glossary

Allophone A phonetic realisation. The manner in which a phoneme varies subject to the influence of, for example, adjacent phones.

Anarthria Complete inability to articulate sounds. Both voice and resonance are affected. Neuropathological in origin. Dysarthria is a less severe form.

Angular gyrus The posterior part of the parietal lobe of the brain concerned with the integration of sensory input.

Broca's area Anterior area of the cerebral cortex concerned with the planning and organisation of speech.

Cerebellum Part of the brain that regulates and modifies movement through input from sensory pathways and through its connections with subcortical and cortical areas.

Diadochokinesis In speech, is the inability to carry out rapid alternating and repetitive movements of the articulatory organs.

Dysarthria See Anarthria.

Gilles de la Tourette syndrome A neurological condition characterised by involuntary tics, both facial and vocal, expiratory noises, echolalia.

Haptic perception That which derives from tactile and proprioceptive input.

Hyperlexia Abnormally advanced reading ability without necessarily understanding the content.

Illocution A term used in speech act theory; that which involves the speaker directly, e.g. thanking, promising, describing. Compare perlocution where the speaker's utterance has an effect upon the listener. Note: Piagetian theory uses this term to denote action accompanying verbalisation.

Lexicon The store of linguistic knowledge concerning structural properties of a language.

Logogens Lexical stores. A logogen collects information relating to the word it stores via perceptual pathways. It is connected both to the semantic/cognitive system enabling meaning to be accessed and to the response system so that the appropriate word may be produced.

Metalinguistics The study of awareness of the properties of language.

Metathesis In linguistics, a change in the sequence of sounds, syllables or words within an utterance, e.g. spoonerisms.

Morpheme The smallest functional unit of language relating to the composition of words.

Myelin A protective covering for the nerve fibres. Its presence facilitates speed of transmission. Myelination of certain nerve pathways is a maturational feature.

Organ of Corti A sensory part of the cochlea of the ear. The function of its receptors is to convert sound pressure waves into electrical impulses that are transmitted via the eighth cranial nerve to the brain. See Medial geniculate body.

Paradigmatic response In psycholinguistics, a term used to describe associated responses to a stimulus word. Paradigmatic responses are in the same word class, e.g. cake–bread–biscuit. Compare Syntagmatic.

Phonology The study of contrastive sound systems within a specific language.

Pragmatics A linguistic term that describes the study of the way in which language is used in social interaction.

Proprioception Awareness of movements of the body, in this context with special reference to movements within the vocal tract (also Kinaesthesia).

Prosody The melody of a language determined by non-segmental features of pitch, stress, loudness and timing.

Reticular system A network of nuclei and fibres within the medulla oblongata. One of its functions is to maintain appropriate levels of muscular tension throughout the body including the vocal tract.

Semantics The study of the meaning of language.

Supplementary motor cortex An area on the medial surface of the cerebral hemisphere adjacent to the motor and somaesthetic strips. Its function may be concerned with the timing and sequential aspects of speech production.

Syntagmatic In psycholinguistics an associated response involving a different word category, e.g. bed–sleep–dream.

Syntax The study of the way in which words relate to one another in a language.

Taxonomy Classification and categorisation, e.g. parts of speech.

Tone The syllable within a tone on which a change of pitch occurs.

Tone group A stretch of speech extending from six to eight syllables having one prominent tone, the nuclear stress.

Tonicity The syllable within a tone unit that carries maximum stress.

Visispeech Instrumentation that records and displays on a screen, intonation and stress patterns generated by a speaker.

Vocable Babble used meaningfully.

Subject Index

Author Index

245